Easy Steps

to

CORRECT

SPEECH

A Mini-book for Self-Improvement

IDA R. BELLEGARDE

HARLO PRESS   DETROIT, MICH.

DEDICATION

*To my captive audience—the students in my classes
at the Agricultural, Mechanical, and Normal college—
this book is lovingly dedicated.*

Printed By
Harlo Press, 16721 Hamilton, Detroit, Mich. 48203

FOREWORD

This is not a comprehensive text on pronunciation but only a handbook to clear up the rough spots in your speech. If you are speaking American English well enough that you are never in doubt as to your pronunciation and use of words, if you are always sure that your use of language is Standard English, and if you are sure that you will not be accused of using substandard English, this book is not for you.

But if you are, at times, uncertain of the proper use of certain common expressions and pronunciations this book will help you to quickly and easily clear up weaknesses in your speech.

It is not necessary to remind you what the power of speech can mean to you. Speech power is communication at its best. Correct speech is absolutely necessary for advancement in any field; and it can be acquired easily and rapidly through a dedicated effort. Any advancement today hinges on how well you use the English language. Your ability to think, and to express your thoughts, depends on your pronunciation and the type and size of the vocabulary you develop.

The importance of clear speech cannot be overemphasized. It is the key to success, an open sesame to a whole new, wonderful world. If you will spend a few moments each day earnestly practicing your exercises you will be richly rewarded far beyond your wildest dreams. Once you become accustomed to your daily routine it will become more and more pleasurable; and you will discover that you are lengthening your study periods because of the pleasure you are getting from studying. You will awake some night to find that you have been practicing your exercises in your sleep. Then, you've got it made! Your success is assured.

Other "Mini-books in preparation are: *Easy Steps To Good Grammar, and Easy Steps to a Large Vocabularly,* Volumes I, II, and III.

IDA R. BELLEGARDE
A.M.&N. College
Pine Bluff, Arkansas

TABLE OF CONTENTS

THINGS TO REMEMBER

1. While practicing your exercises, overemphasize the sound of the letters or words that you are studying so that you can distinctly *hear* the sound.

2. Exaggerate the movements of your tongue, lips, and teeth so that you can distinctly *feel* the sound as well as hear it.

3. Use a hand mirror so that you can *see* the difference in the production of the sounds, as well as to hear and feel the difference.

4. Begin slowly until you are sure of the pronunciation, then speed up the repetition until you are speaking at normal speed.

5. In consonant combinations, you should blend the two sounds so closely that they lose their separate identities and merge into a single sound.

6. There are two types of speech sounds: voiced sounds, and voiceless, or whispered sounds. Voiced sounds are made with a murmur or a hum; voiceless sounds are whispered.

7. All practice periods must be done *aloud.*

8. Exaggerate your speech *only* in practice. Overemphasis of the speech sounds results in stilted speech, which is considered improper by today's standards.

9. Good speech is a matter of practice. Drill. Drill. Drill.

Chapter 1

THE SOUNDS OF ENGLISH

A knowledge of English sounds will clear up most of your speech faults. To speak well you must use your tongue, teeth, and lips properly. Many students are guilty of being lip-lazy. Lip-laziness is a serious offense, and you should work hard to correct this malady.

THE CONSONANT SOUNDS

The Sound of P

How to Produce P: P is a whispered sound. It is made by pressing the lips together, then forcing them apart with the breath.

Practice the *p* sound by repeating the following, making *only* the sound:

p,p,p, p,p,p, p,p,p, p,p,p, p,p,p

Repeat the following ten times:

pay, pea, pie, po, poo, pu;   pay, pea, pie, po, poo, pu

people, purple, ample, staple, dapple, dimple, rumple, crumple

rip, tap, cap, lap, sap, map, nap, dap, gap, rap, dope, soap, elope

The Sound of B

How to Produce B: B is a voiced sound, that is, you must make a slight sound with your voice when producing it. Press the lips together as you did for *p,* then force them apart while making a slight murmur.

Practice the *b* sound by repeating the following, making only the sound:

b,b,b,   b,b,b,   b,b,b,   b,b,b,   b,b,b

Repeat the following ten times:

bay, bee, by, bo, boo, bu;   bay, bee, by, bo, boo, bu

dabble, dibble, double, amble, ramble, crumble, tumble, scramble,

tab, cab, lab, crab, nab, rib, grub, stub, bob, cub, rub, dab

Practice the difference between *b* and *p* by repeating aloud the following word pairs. Always exaggerate your speech while practicing, so that you can feel the sound as well as hear it.

pat, bat   plead, bleed   clapper, clabber

put, but   peer, beer   dapper, dabber

pack, back   pair, bare   staple, stable

patch, batch   paid, blade   ample, amble

park, bark   peck, beck   flappy, flabby

Repeat aloud the following ten times:

1. The people watched with pleasure the beauty of sail-boats proudly unfurling their sails in the placid Pacific bay.

2. The puppy rode on the back of the prancing pony.

3. She stood primly preening herself before a mirror.

4. The bubbling and babbling of the boiling kettle caused the puppy to become playful.

5. He ambled down the broad road that was dappled in sunshine and shadow.

6. Paul went promptly to pick blueberries in the berry patch.

7. Blueberries bloom in a basket behind Barbara's bicycle.

8. The busy bustling harbor brought to mind the plight of the poor people back home.

The Sound of D

How to Produce D: D is a voiced sound and is formed by pressing the front of the tongue (*not the tip*) against the upper gums, then expelling the breath while making a murmuring sound.

Note: For our purpose, the front of the tongue is the part next to the tip.

Practice the *d* sound by repeating the following, making only the sound:

d,d,d,   d,d,d,   d,d,d,   d,d,d,   d,d,d

Repeat the following ten times, exaggerating the *d* sound:

day, dee, daw, doe, doo;   day, dee, daw, doe, doo

day, dog, dam, dime, door, down, maiden, ladder, bedding

leader, hidden, radish, lid, mad, hand, yard, child, reward

1. The dog was dozing while Dan dabbled in the ditch.
2. The debt was paid the day the deductions were made.
3. Dora delved deeply into the data and diagrammed it for Diahann.
4. It is degrading to delight in delusions.
5. The detour directed us through a deserted desert.

The T and D Sounds

Do not substitute *t* for *d*. In substandard speech the letters *t* and *d* are often substituted for each other. This type of substitution sets a person apart as being illiterate and should be avoided like a plague. To guard against this type of substitution, repeat the following pairs of words aloud ten times:

dent, tent   little, ladle   sat, sad

dip, tip   lit, lid   latter, ladder

Dan, tan   colt, cold   petal, peddle

den, ten   mutter, mudder   heat, heed

dime, time   metal, medal   bolt, bold

duck, tuck   late, laid   taffy, daffy

The Sound of F

How to Produce F: F is a whispered sound, that is, you do not use the voice to produce it. It is formed by placing the lower lip against the upper teeth, and forcing the breath quickly through the space between the teeth and lip.

Practice drill:

f,f,f,   f,f,f,   f,f,f,   f,f,f,   f,f,f

Repeat the following aloud ten times, exaggerating the *f* sound:

fee, fi, fo, foo, fay, fum;   fee, fi, fo, foo, fay, fum

file, fail, for, found, fun, offer, buffer, duffer, loafer, saffron

scaffold, drafted, proof, surf, brief, leaf, laugh, cough, puff, fluff

The F and V Sounds

The letters *f* and *v* are often confused. Do not say *leaf* for *leave.*

The Sound of V

How to Produce V: V is a voiced sound. It is made by placing the lower lip gently *against the front of the upper front teeth,* allowing a small overlap. Now, force the breath through the teeth while *sliding* the lip down and back from the teeth, and making a slight murmuring sound. Practice the *v* sound until you can do it smoothly, allowing the sound to trail off.

Practice drill:

v,v,v,   v,v,v,   v,v,v,   v,v,v,   v,v,v

Repeat the following aloud ten times, using a mirror to watch your lips.

vay, vee, vi, vo, voo, vue;   vay, vee, vi, vo, voo, vue

vane, van, vale, very, vend, viper, vest, serve, wave, grieve, five

prove, love, quiver, liver, cover, ravage, cavity, gravity, avian

grief, grieve   fine, vine   loafer, lover

sheaf, sheave   face, vase   reference, reverence

leaf, leave   raffle, ravel   ferry, very

surf, serve   offer, over   plaintiff, plaintive

fail, vale   surface, service   shuffle, shovel

1. The veterans of foreign wars have a fierce concern for the disclosure of facts in the field of foreign affairs.

2. The development of true friendship can be fatal to romantic love.

3. A free exchange of views is very necessary for friendly communication.

4. Every father dreams of fame for his family.

The Sound of G as in Go (hard g)

Note: Soft g, as in gem and age is pronounced like j.

How to Produce *g* as in Go: G, as in go, is a voiced sound. Press the back of the tongue against the soft palate, then expel the breath with an explosive murmur, but with slightly less breath force than for K.

Practice drill:

g,g,g,   g,g,g,   g,g,g,   g,g,g,   g,g,g

Repeat the following aloud ten times, exaggerating the *g* sound:

gah, gay, gaw, go, goo;   gah, gay, gaw, go, goo

gay, gold, guest, gulls, guide, girdle, gurgle, frigate, giggle

agony, bugle, rugged, beg, dog, lag, clog, vague, egg

1. The governor gazed at the gifted girls giggling in the buggy.

2. The frog leaped over the log to get away from the dog.

3. The girls giggled at the boys who wore goggles.

The Sound of H

How to Produce H: H is a whispered sound. Curve the sides of the tongue against the upper jaw teeth, making a groove along the midline. Build up the breath and expel it forcefully above the upper gum ridge.

Practice drill:

h,h,h,   *h,h,h,*   *h,h,h,*   *h,h,h,*   *h,h,h*

Repeat the following aloud ten times, exaggerating the *h* sound:

he, hay, hen, hum, her, how, abhor, ahoy, behind, inhuman, inhumane,

inhale, uphold, hail, ahead, behalf, behave, grasshopper, inhabit,

mohair, perhaps, prohibit, rehearse, hero

1. The haughty horse held his head high when Henry rode happily by.

2. Her rehearsal was hampered by Helen who happened to be passing by.

3. Her husband hurried down the hall as he made a hasty exit.

4. Hilda was happy to hide the hound to keep Harry from hunting.

The Sound of J

How to Pronounce J: J is a voiced sound. Press the *front* of the tongue firmly against the upper gum ridge, and the sides firmly against the upper jaw teeth. Build up the breath, then release it suddenly and forcefully.

Practice drill (Make sound only):

j,j,j,   j,j,j,   j,j,j,   j,j,j,   j,j,j

Repeat aloud the following ten times, exaggerating the *j* sound:

jeer, jar, gem, jam, germ, journey, edged, reject, agent, raging,

religion, injury, hedge, urge, fudge, bridge, sage, courage

1. The raging sea injured the religious agent who had been encouraged to make the journey.

2. The judge made the journey in January.

3. The jury judiciously ruled against the juggler who injured Johnny's jugular vein.

4. Juvenile jazzmen played jazz before a jaundiced audience.

The Sound of K

How to Produce K: K is a whispered sound. Press the back of the tongue against the hard palate, build up the breath, then force the tongue away suddenly and forcefully.

Practice drill:

k,k,k,   k,k,k,   k,k,k,   k,k,k,   k,k,k

Repeat the following aloud ten times, exaggerating the *k* sound:

call, cool, car, kit, picnic, care, echo, school, ache, escape, lock

American, neck, sick, lack, nook, duck, kind, skunk, scheme, thank

1. The cluster of conversational furniture gave a cluttered appearance to a contemporary conventional room.

2. The kite quickly climbed the skyway through the scudding clouds.

3. He kindly considered to concern himself about conditions in the colonies.

The Sound of L

How to Produce the Sound of L: L is a voiced sound, formed by placing the tip of the tongue lightly against the upper gums, but with both sides lowered to permit the escape of the breath. Release the breath while making a murmuring sound.

Exercise drill:

l,l,l l,l,l, l,l,l l,l,l, l,l,l

Repeat aloud the following ten times, exaggerating the *l* sound:

lay, lark, let, look, learn, loon, alley, olive, silver, island

eleven, delight, will, shall, tell, scholar, school, shovel, annual

1. Ladies languished on the leeward side of the limping launch.

2. Laughing wavelets lulled water lilies lying on the surface of the lake.

3. The little old lamp lighter filled the pail with olive oil.

4. We looked in the alley by lamp light for eleven little limpkins.

5. Lola believed Lloyd when he told her that she looked like a living doll.

6. Anti-air pollution falls within the realm of new ideals.

7. The cultural upheaval will result in the removal of large segments of the population.

The Sound of M

How to Produce M: M is a nasal sound, that is, the sound must come through the nose instead of the mouth. Press the lips together as for P, then make a humming sound while expelling the breath through the nose.

Practice drill:

m,m,m,   m,m,m,   m,m,m,   m,m,m,   m,m,m

Repeat aloud the following ten times exaggerating the *m* sound:

many, meek, more, mouse, move, mule, my, among, coming, common

lamb, loom, seem, tame, lamp, tramp, slumped, romps, sums, overwhelm

1. My mother baked mince pies on summer mornings.
2. Many music lovers may find happiness beside murmuring streams in the summertime.
3. The criticism of his patriotism was the result of his optimism.
4. Her witticism resulted in the criticism of her enthusiasm.
5. Mamie was hemming the summer skimmer.
6. The romper set tramped through the room overwhelming the women.

The Sound of N

How to Produce N: Press the tip of the tongue against the upper gum ridge, and the sides of the tongue against the upper jaw teeth, to block the air passage at the sides. Expel the breath through the nose while making a humming sound.

Exercise drill:

n,n,n,   n,n,n,   n,n,n,   n,n,n,   n,n,n

Repeat aloud the following ten times, exaggerating the *n* sound:

none, never, neither, night, nature, nowhere, natural, normal

inner, beginning, internal, handsome, fantasy, hinder, sandal

intern, offend, begin, attention, assassin, sinner, scant

1. Neighbors are never numerous in time of need.

2. Many mothers never worry when their newest apron is neatly torn.

3. Neither Nora nor the nurse remained neutral about the dance.

4. A branch from a juniper landed on a bunch of ferns.

The Sound of R

How to Produce the Sound of R: Curve the tip of the tongue backward toward the roof of the mouth, but without touching. Now, expel the breath while making a murmuring sound.

Drill exercise:

r,r,r,   r,r,r,   r,r,r   r,r,r   r,r,r

Repeat aloud the following ten times, exaggerating the *r* sound:

ray, raw, rat, run, rare, ruin, throw, freeze, dream, shrank, train, prince, errand, every, very, hurry, sorry, serene, carbon, perform,

arrow, orange, eastern, southern, strangle, script, shrimp, stars

1. The fragrance of roses was rampant in the morning breeze.

2. The hurricane winds were pregnant with freezing rain.

3. Robert preferred red wine and French bread to a roast beef dinner.

4. Scurring rain clouds hurried to the north before a breeze that did not touch the earth.

5. The rolling currents in the rampaging river released torrents of water.

6. A religious regime that restricts liberty is frequently refused by the congregation.

The Sound of S

How to Produce S: S is a whispered sound, and requires careful adjustment of tongue and teeth. Place the sides of the tongue against the upper jaw teeth with sides curved upward, and place the tip of the tongue against the lower gums below the lower teeth. This creates a groove along the mid-line of the tongue. Now, expel the breath in a soft hissing sound *against the cutting edges of the lower teeth.*

Drill exercise:

s,s,s,   s,s,s,   s,s,s,   s,s,s,   s,s,s

Repeat aloud the following ten times, exaggerating the *s* sound:

sink, sum, sought, sip, seal, soft, muscle, mistake, mystery, muscadine, fascinate, custom, pass, miss, moss, ice, race, bus,

sing, kiss, last, cloves, waves, strive, gasoline, doves, pshaw

1. The silent silver sea glistened under the slanting moonbeams
2. We would all like to be on the side of success.
3. The silence was broken only by the swish of waves on the seashore.
4. Waves swirled around the sinking ship.
5. The sound of singing sifted through the shining shrubs.
6. Susie selected Sylvia to secure a strong sash that would remain secure.

The Sound of Z

How to Produce the Z Sound: Place the sides of the tongue against the upper jaw teeth, curving upward, and the tip of the tongue against the lower gums. Bring the upper and lower teeth almost together, then expel the breath between the teeth while making a buzzing sound.

Note: Z is represented by *x* at the beginning of words, as in *xylophone* and *xerox*. The *z* sound is sometime used for *s* when it falls within the middle of a word, such as: *absorb, absurd, desolate, greasy, museum,* and *measels.*

Drill exercise:

z,z,z,   z,z,z,   z,z,z,   z,z,z,   z,z,z

Learn the difference between *z* and *s* pronouncing the following pairs of words. Be sure to stress the hissing sound of *s.*

zeal, seal   his, hiss

zoo, Sioux   eyes, ice

zinc, sink   rays, race

zipper, sipper   buzzing, busing

fizzy, fussy   lazy, lacey

face, phaze   price, prize

peace, peas   muscle, muzzle

loose, lose   race, raze

mace, maize   grace, graze

Repeat aloud the following ten times, exaggerating the z sound:

1. Some zebras belong in a zoo; others on the football field.

2. The lazy, grazing cattle were pleasing to the eyes.

3. The buzzing bees were dazed and dozed in the tubs.

4. Zesty smells fell from the busy trees bending in the hazy skies.

The Sound of T

How to Produce T: Press the tip of the tongue against the upper gums, behind the upper teeth (*but do not touch the teeth*), then force the tongue away with the whispered breath.

Repeat the *t* sound in the following:

t,t,t,   t,t,t,   t,t,t,   t,t,t,   t,t,t

Repeat the following aloud ten times, exaggerating the *t* sound:

tan, tin, time, tune, tall, bottle, pattern, little, letter
better, habit, polite, excite, forget, regret, water, center
bottom, beetles, putter, sitter, pity, beating, utter, dating

1. She was in the habit of forgetting little courtesies.
2. It is better to write the letter on the table.
3. Thomas showed tact in tackling the troublesome problem.
4. The teakettle sat on a table made of teakwood.
5. Ten tall tailors taught the entire class.
6. The tall timbers of Timbuktu appeared to touch the sky.
7. Little Rock is noted for its interest in artistic accomplishments.
8. The pattern and buttons for the winter coat were put into the basket.

The Sound of W

To Make the W Sound: Place the tip of the tongue behind the lower front teeth, and purse the lips as if to whistle. Make a slight humming sound as you let your breath *flow* easily through the opening.

Drill exercise:

w,w,w,   w,w,w,   w,w,w,   w,w,w,   w,w,w

Repeat the following aloud ten times, exaggerating the *w* sound:

walk, west, wear, willow, water, wings, awake, aware, reward,

whirlwind, waterway, wail, wear, weigh, wish, wine, worse,

wool, wood, always, forward, upward, onward, dwindle, language

1. The woman filled the wheelbarrow with wildflowers as she walked along the highway.

2. The wailing of the winter wind whistled through the weatherbeaten structure.

3. The window washer worked well in the swirling whirlwind.

4. If you are willing to watch the words you use, you will be rewarded.

5. The memory of walking homeward through wild wintry winds weighed on his mind.

6. Wee Willie reported that a wicked wild witch sat in the weeping willows.

7. Winds wailed and whimpered in the whispering willows.

The Sound of X

How to Pronounce X: X is a whispered sound and is produced by blending the sounds *k* and *s* together. Press the back of the tongue against the roof of the mouth, as for *k*, then blend it into the hissing sound of *s*.

Note: X, at the beginning of a word is pronounced like *z*, as in Xerxes, xerox, Xenophon, Xavier, xylophone.

Repeat the sounds of the following:

k,s,   k,s,   k,s,   k,s,   k,s,   k,s,   k,s,

ks,   ks,   ks,   ks,   ks,   ks,   ks,   ks

Repeat aloud the following ten times, exaggerating the *x* sound:

exit, sexton, vexed, excite, expect, excellent, books, locks, fix

coax, flax, antiques, annex, bedecks, circumflex, complex, convex

multiplex, reflex, perplex, sex, affects, architects, exceed, excel

1. He rightfully expected excellent marks for extra work.

2. Max was vexed at the sexton for expecting him to coax sixty hours of extra work from his books.

3. He fixed the locks after the exit of oxen from the field of flax.

4. The executive expected the architects to erect a complex annex.

5. Her excellent and exciting rendition was excessively acclaimed.

6. They made an exhaustive examination with an exaggerated air of importance.

7. The exotic perfume was an exhilarating influence in creating a feeling of exaltation.

8. The exhibit was an example of what an executive can create with twigs and eggs.

9. He was exempted from an exorbitant fee charged by an exacting accountant.

10. Exotic flowers clung to the logs exhibiting an auxiliary prop for the scene.

The Sound of Y, as in You

How to Produce Y: Y, as in you, is a whispered sound. Lift the middle of the tongue toward the roof of the mouth, allowing the sides of the tongue to press against the upper jaw teeth, as for long *e,* then expel the breath up and out.

Drill exercise:

y,y,y,   y,y,y,   y,y,y,   y,y,y,   y,y,y

Repeat the following aloud ten times, exaggerating the *y* sound:

you, yard, yield, yen, youth, year, union, onion, picayune, opinion beyond, canyon, yet, lawyer, yeast, yesterday, vineyard, yak

million, yours, genial, year, young, companion

1. Yesterday you were yearning to go beyond the canyon for the reunion.

2. You saw the youth in the yard yelling at the Union officer.

3. It is Daniel's opinion that the yield of the onion crop will go beyond yesterday's.

4. The youth yearned to return to civilian life.

5. A congenial civilian raised spaniels for a useful livelihood.

Chapter 2

THE CONSONANT COMBINATIONS

In pronouncing the consonant combinations, you must blend the two sounds so well that they lose their separate identities and merge into a single sound.

The Ch Combination

To Make the Ch Sound: Press the tip of the tongue firmly against the upper gum ridge with sides pressed firmly against the upper teeth, and build up a column of air under pressure. Then, release the breath suddenly and rapidly.

Practice drill:

ch,ch,ch, ch,ch,ch, ch,ch,ch, ch,ch,ch, ch,ch,ch

Repeat the following aloud ten times, exaggerating the *ch* sound:

church, chart, chapter, cheat, chimes, chair, check, child, choose

bachelor, coaching, etching, itching, matching, catcher, merchant

touch, pitch, batch, rich, latch, notch, research, smirch, perch

1. The chimes from the church tower were heard above the churning of the waves.
2. The sea urchins brought by the merchants caused a chain reaction of itching.

3. The mischievous children chased the chickens into the church.

4. The chimpanzee watched for a chance to filch the watch.

5. The etching was placed on a chair and checked by the chief coach.

The Sh Consonant Combination

How to Make the Sh Sound: Place the tip of the tongue against the lower gums below the lower teeth, and the sides of the tongue pressed against the upper teeth. Expel the whispered breath through slightly protruding lips.

Drill on the following, making only the sound:

sh,sh,sh,   sh,sh,sh,   sh,sh,sh,   sh,sh,sh,   sh,sh,sh

Repeat the following ten times, exaggerating the *sh* sound:

she, shade, shell, shut, share, shower, shall, shine, shoe, shop

ashen, bishop, cushion, motion, ocean, pension, tension, usher

fish, slush, bush, dash, squash, crash, fresh, mesh, push, mush

1. The children enjoyed splashing in the ocean and gathering sea shells while on their vacation.

2. She shared fresh fish with Felicia after it was washed and placed in a dish.

3. She heard a sharp shuffling noise when she called to the boys to shovel the snow from the shed.

4. She shouted that the dishes were mashing the fish.

5. The shiftless shoeshine boy set up shop at the fresh fish market.

The Zh Consonant Combination

The *zh* sound is a voiced sound. Place the tip of the tongue *below the lower gums*, and the sides of the tongue between the upper and lower jaw teeth. Expel the breath between the teeth while making a buzzing sound.

Practice drill:

zh,zh,zh,   zh,zh,zh,   zh,zh,zh,   zh,zh,zh   zh,zh,zh

Repeat the following aloud ten times, exaggerating the *zh* sound:

> rouge, beige, leisure, osier, allusion, glaciers, closure, measure
> azure, cortege, seisure, lesion, mirage, illusion, invasion
>
> camouflage, prestige, barrage, corsage, sabotage, garage, usual

1. Her prestige was enhanced by her decisions on leisure-time features.
2. Her beige corsage was camouflaged by an illusion.
3. It was his pleasure to convey the decision of the closure of their activities.
4. The illusion of leisure in the garage was merely a mirage.
5. His delusions of grandeur resulted in the invasion and seizure of the whole army.

The St Combination

How to Produce the *St* Sound: The best way to make the *st* sound is to blend the two separate sounds. Turn back and review the production of the two sounds, then, drill on the following:

s,s,s,   t,t,t,   s,s,s,   t,t,t,   s,s,s,   t,t,t

s,t,   s,t,   s,t,   s,t,   s,t,   s,t,   s,t

st,st,st,   st,st,st,   st,st,st,   st,st,st

Repeat the following aloud, exaggerating the *st* sound:

stay, start, step, stout, stair, vest, must, first, least, roast

tossed, missed, pressed, asked, face, passed, dressed, zest

just, cost, stringent, plastic, substitution, astounding

1. The student studied the statues of the statesmen in the rotunda.

2. Students of political science are required to study the statutes of the state.

3. The books on state law were stashed in the State-house.

Note: The *st* sound will be reviewed further in the section on "Combinations at the Beginning of Words."

Th as in Thick

Th, as in thick, is a whispered sound and is made by placing the tip of the tongue between the front teeth, and expelling the breath quickly. Repeat the following aloud ten times, exaggerating the *th* sound:

theme, thimble, thumb, thick, theory, thousand, method, pith

wealthy, author, panther, pathetic, path, health, Smith, with

teeth, truth, earth, mirth, myth, strength, length, month, worth

1. He thought a thousand times about the threat of ill health facing him.

2. The author used his own method in writing the theme.

3. The wealthy blacksmith planted a path thick with thistles.

4. Three panthers stalked through a thicket of thorn trees.

5. The thumping of thunder was heard throughout the night.

Note: In substandard speech, other sounds are often substituted for the *th* sound. This type of substitution is considered illiterate and ignorant and should be strictly avoided.

Do not substitute F for th

This substitution is the biggest offender, and sets its user apart as being very illiterate. Its most frequent occurrence is at the end of words, though it also appears at the beginning.

Repeat aloud ten times, the following word pairs and exaggerate the *th* sound:

Say:

with, not *wif*   *birth,* not *birf*

teeth, not *teef*   *truth,* not *truf*

Smith, not *Smiff*   *north,* not *norf*

wreath, not *reef*   *worth,* not *worf*

mouth, not *mouf*   *both,* not *bof*

thin, not *fin*   *thought,* not *fought*

three, not *free*   *thresh,* not *fresh*

Do not substitute t for th

Say:

thank, not *tank*   *think,* not *tink*

thought, not *taught*   *thin,* not *tin*

thick, not *tick*   *theme,* not *teem*

Th as in They

Th as in *they* is a voiced sound. Place the tip of the tongue between the front teeth and gently blow while making a buzzing sound.

Drill exercise:

they, thee, thy, tho, thoo;   they, thee, thy, tho, thoo

Repeat the following aloud ten times, exaggerating the *th* sound:

this, them, they, that, than, though, thatch, theater, thing

aesthetic, author, athlete, ether, mothy, youthful, either

neither, bother, weather, soothe, writhe, blithe, teethe

1. They thought that they would bathe in the thermal bath.
2. The weather prevented the thieves from taking the clothing.
3. The angry youths were soothed by the stormy weather that slithered around them.
4. Farther and farther they rode, wondering whether they would be able to tether their horses.
5. The feathers were blown hither and thither by the blithering wind that blithely blew in writhing circles.

Do not substitute V for Th

Say:

clothe, not *clove*   *breathe,* not *breve*

those, not *vose*   *further,* not *fervor*

bathe, not *bave*   *teethe,* not *teeve*

wreathe, not *wreve*   *smoothed,* not *smooved*

Do not substitute D for Th

Say:

this, not *dis*   *they,* not *day*

them, not *dem*   *though,* not *doe*

with, not *wid*   *there,* not *dare*

The Wh Sound

The *wh* sound is a whispered sound. Place the tip of the tongue behind the lower front teeth, and purse the lips as if to whistle. Then, expel the breath quickly and hard, as if to blow out a match.

Drill exercise:

wh,wh,wh,   wh,wh,wh,   wh,wh,wh,
wh,wh,wh,   wh,wh,wh

Repeat the following aloud ten times, exaggerating the *wh* sound:

whale, what wheel, when, where, which, whimper, whisper, whistle

anywhere, awhile, bewhiskered, bobwhite, elsewhere, meanwhile,

1. The wild whimpering wind whispered and whined through the wilderness.

2. We wondered where we were going as we wandered through the winding waterway.

3. The wind whistled as the millwheel whirled.

4. A whiffling wind whimpered among the trees and somewhere a bobwhite whistled.

5. The whale wheeled and whirled, whipping its tail in the white salt spray.

6. The whirling old wagon wheel wheezed to a whining stop.

Chapter 3

THE BASIC VOWEL SOUNDS

How Vowel Sounds Differ
from Consonant Sounds

1. Consonant sounds are made by restricting the flow of air with the tongue, teeth or lips; vowels are made by an unrestricted flow of air out of the mouth.

2. Vowels constitute families of sounds: the *e* family, the *a* family, the *o* family, the *i* family, and the *u* family.

3. The different vowel sounds are made by altering the shape of the mouth, or by altering the position of the tongue.

4. All vowel sounds are made with the voice. They are never voiceless; some consonant sounds are voiceless, or whispered.

5. The tongue and lower jaw are very important in producing vowel sounds. You must pay particular attention to the formation of the tongue: whether it is bunched toward the front of the mouth, the middle of the mouth, or the back of the mouth. The humping, or bunching, or arching of the tongue makes an important difference.

6. In the production of the vowel sound, in almost every case, the tip of the tongue is placed against the lower teeth.

THE VOWEL FAMILIES

The A Family

a as in fate, ape, (long a)

a as in fat, lap, ask, am, at, (short a)

ä as in car, father

a as in ago, has the same sound of *e* in agent; *i,* in sanity; *o,* in comply; and *u,* in focus. For our purpose, we shall call this vowel sound a "short-short *u.*"

The A Family

a, as in Late

How to Produce *a* As in Late: Long *a* requires movement of the tongue as well as positioning. With the sides of the tongue against the upper jaw teeth, slightly arch the back of the tongue toward the roof of the mouth. With the lips parted and drawn slightly back, expel the breath with a murmur while moving your arched tongue a little higher toward the roof of the mouth.

Repeat the following aloud ten times:

abe, able, ace, ache, acorn, age, aid, aim, ape, Asia, ate

babe, bail, base, dale, daze, face, fade, guage, great, safe

bay, day, fray, gay, hay, jay, weigh, they, stray, stay

1. The horses neighed and ate hay while jaybirds stayed in the bay.

2. The veils faded under a great and blazing sun.

3. The tape was safe in a pail when the raid was staged.

4. He faced the gaze of gay ailing men as a May rain fell.

a, As in Fat

How to Produce *a* As in Fat: Place the tip of the tongue behind the lower front teeth and raise the back of the tongue slightly toward the back of the roof, an expel the breath while making a murmuring sound.

Repeat the following aloud ten times:

act, add, after, altitude, am, ample, animal, ant, anthem, apple

band, fad, graduate, had, hat, lack, rack, sang, sat, tack, pat

mattress, pat, path, sack, sallow, Sally, satire, landing, lad

1. The actual act came after the hat landed on the lad.
2. Sally sang a satire and sat down on a sack.
3. Allen had to haggle over his animal and ant act.
4. Apples are apt to become a fad with the graduates.

a, As in Father

How to Produce *a* As in Father: This sound is made by placing the tip of the tongue behind the lower front teeth, and relaxing and flattening the tongue. With your mouth opened wide, release the breath with a humming sound.

Repeat the following aloud ten times:

alms, aria, ark, obstacle, obstinate, octopus, odd, ominous, on

balm, bar, car, father, opera, opportune, cod, cot, palm, rock

ah, aha, bah, bourgeois, faux pas, mamma, Shah, spa, Utah

1. Father was calm when the swan wandered into the yard.
2. The bourgeois was accused of committing a faux pas.
3. The clock rocked on the dock when the obstinate octopus was caught.
4. Sergeant Tom remained calm when the guard dropped a bomb on his car.

The E Family

e, As in Eve

How to Produce *e* As in Eve: Place the tip of the tongue behind the lower front teeth, and bunche the front of the tongue toward the front of the roof of the mouth while pressing the sides against the upper jaw teeth. With mouth slightly open and lips slightly spread, expel the breath with a murmuring sound.

Practice drill:

e,e,e,   e,e,e,   e,e,e,   e,e,e,   e,e,e

Repeat the following aloud ten times:

each, eager, ease, ego, eagle, easel, easy, beat, cheat

cheese, feast, feel, zeal, meat, seek, agree, be, fee, reed

free, he, key, sea, knee, eager, conceited, weaned, speak, leak

1. The eager beaver gleefully eats the fleeing eel.
2. Each eagle feels free to feed on a meal of yeasty cheese.
3. He seeks to cheat the dealer but has agreed to go easy on the deal.
4. She dreams and schemes eagerly as she feeds meal to her weaver.
5. The water seemed to seep through the peeling seams.

e, As in Let

How to Produce *e,* As in Let: Place the tip of the tongue behind the lower front teeth, slightly arch the middle of the tongue toward the middle of the roof of the mouth, and with the sides of the tongue pressed against the upper jaw teeth expel the breath with a murmuring sound.

Repeat the following aloud ten times:

ebony, echo, edible, edit, egg, ensign, exercise, epoch, bell, deck, fell

head, hen, tent, yell, said, edge, effigy, elbow, elephant, elf, elm

end, entrance, epoch, exit

1. The red-headed ensign wrecked the car at a dead-end road.
2. The editor read well in bed instead of in the tent.
3. Ten men mended their ways after they fell in the well.
4. The bell was welded on the deck of the red ship.
5. Fred has wed a second belle after he shed the red-head.

er, As in Over

How to Produce *er,* As in Over: The front (not the tip) of the tongue should be raised and curled back slightly toward the roof of the mouth, the mouth slightly rounded and tensed, while expelling the breath with a murmur.

Practice the *u* and *r* sounds separately, then blend them together:

u,u,u,   r,r,r,   u,u,u,   r,r,r,   u,u,u,   r,r,r,   u,u,u,   r,r,r

u,r,   u,r,   u,r,   u,r,   u,r,   u,r,   u,r,   u,r

ur,   ur,   ur,   ur,   ur,   ur,   ur,   ur

Repeat the following aloud ten times, exaggerating the *er* sound:

early, earnest, err, erstwhile, urban, urge, birch, bird, hurt heard, purse, worth, blur, confer, her, fur, prefer, over

under, catcher, water, father, never, heavier, brighter, blinker

1. The blinker on his tractor was brighter than his brother's.

2. The cover over the silver was lighter and shorter.

3. Water in the summer is better for swimmers than in the winter.

4. Sooner or later her sister will get thinner and prettier.

The I Family

i, As in Bite

How to Produce *i* As in Bite: Long *i* requires tongue movement as well as positioning. Place the tip of the tongue behind the lower front teeth, and bunch the back of the tongue in the back of the mouth. Expel the breath with a murmur while arching the back of the tongue toward the roof of the mouth.

Repeat the following aloud ten times:

tie, my, aisle, eye, icicle, island, bite, crime, file, kite

rhyme, buy, fry, try, why, tile, dial, dime, time, dine, mile

ride, height, might, crime, pride, ivory, item, iris, iron

1. Why is it a crime to dine without muscadine wine?

2. The kite flew high over the site of the dry tile.

3. Ida gave a sly sigh and made a try at prying into the item.

4. The bride might have dialed the number in prime time.

5. Mike grew tired and cried when he wasn't hired in time.

i, As in Hit

How to Produce *i* As in Hit: Place the tip of the tongue behind the lower front teeth, and the sides against the upper jaw teeth. Then, arch the front of the tongue toward the roof of the mouth, and expel the breath with a quick murmur.

Repeat the following aloud ten times:

igloo, infant, innocent, inside, itch, mill, hill, big, think

sister, mister, ideology, city, pottery, drowsy, sing, hid

fill, lick, pick, kid, Italian, itch, ditch, insist, initial

1. The innocent infant became ill when it was given a pill.
2. The fish from Italy made a big hit when it was served inside.
3. Bill insisted that his dish was kicked into the pit.
4. Kids and chickens were terror-stricken of the wicked witch.
5. The clicking of the crickets is caused by the friction of prickly feet.

The O Family

o, As in Old

How to Produce the *o* As in Old: Long *o* requires movement of the lips while in production. Place the tip of the tongue behind the lower front teeth, and purse your lips as if to whistle. Arch the back of the tongue toward the soft palate, and expel the breath while making a murmuring sound.

Repeat the following aloud ten times:

oaf, oak, oath, core, ode, only, open, owe, own, ozone, over

boat, coat, coke, hold, loan, loath, rope, soap, sold, stone

crow, dough, foe, go, grow, hoe, low, sew, slow, snow, throw

1. Ozell wrote home for an old coat that had been sold.
2. Joe was told to go home and mow the oats.
3. It is only a stone's throw to the old oak pole.
4. Lola owns the dough that the slow crow stole.
5. The old oak moans and groans as it grows.

o, As in Horn

How to Produce *o* As in Horn: With the lips slightly rounded and protruded, place the tip of the tongue behind the lower front teeth and arch the back of the tongue slightly toward the soft palate, while expelling the breath with a murmur.

Repeat the following aloud ten times:

all, alter, auction, audience, ought, August, author, autumn

applaud, ball, brought, call, caught, fall, fought, gnawed

caw, claw, draw, flaw, gnaw, jaw, law, paw, raw, saw, slaw

1. Maud was caught with the ball that autumn.
2. Authors are often thought to be awed in the presence of an audience.
3. To alter all the flaws, auctions ought to be held in August.

4. The author sought an audition of that awful song.

5. The rats gnawed and clawed the awning before they were caught.

oo, As in Moon

How to Produce the *oo* Sound As in Moon: With lips rounded and protruded, with a small opening, place the tip of the tongue behind the lower front teeth. And with the back of the tongue arched high toward the soft palate, expel the breath with a mooing sound.

Repeat the following aloud ten times:

boom, booth, brute, cool, coop, fool, loop, loot, moon, prove

recruit, snoop, swoop, tooth, youth, bamboo, canoe, cashew

construe, coo, crew, glue, flew, tattoo, through, true, unto

1. Oolong tea is served in Oologah, Oklahoma in the dark of the moon.

2. The women were booed for pulling their oomiack through the boulevard.

3. Soon the booing will stop and the wooing begin.

4. She swooped through the room and threw glue at the kangaroo.

5. Bamboo canoes were glued after they slew the caribou at the zoo.

oo, As in Book

How to Produce the *oo* Sound As in Book: With the lips slightly rounded and protruded, place the tip of the tongue behind the lower front teeth, and arch the back high toward the soft palate. Expel the breath with a low grunt.

Repeat the following aloud ten times:

book, brook, bull, bullet, bully, bush, cook, cooking, could

crook, cushion, should, foot, full, good, hood, hook, look

mistook, nook, overlook, partook, pull, pulley, push, woolen

1. While she cooked she looked for a book in the nook.

2. He should put his foot on the cushion as he pushes the pulley.

3. The sooty pullet overlooked the rook in the woods.

4. We looked at the crook who threw the hook in the brook.

oi, As in Voice

How to Produce the *oi* Sound: The lips should be slightly rounded and slightly protruded. Then, place the tip of the tongue behind the lower front teeth, and arch the back toward the soft palate. But, as you expel the breath with a murmuring sound, arch the front of the tongue toward the roof of the mouth. This movement of the tongue is necessary in making the correct sound.

Practice the sound until you have mastered it, then repeat the following aloud ten times:

oil, ointment, oyster, boil, boys, broil, choice, coil, coin

moist, noise, poise, royal, soil, voice, alloy, annoy, coy,

decoy, deploy, destroy, employ, enjoy, envoy, joy, toy boiler

1. A sailor in an oilskin coat, cried "Ahoy there."

2. A mixture of alloys destroyed the boiler.
3. The boys went fishing for oysters in the roiling river.
4. Her noisy voice annoyed her employer.
5. Joy's voice was the joint choice of Roy and Troy.

ou, As in Out

How to Produce the *ou* Sound: Place the tip of the tongue behind the lower front teeth, with the back relaxed low and flat. Then, while expelling the breath with a murmuring sound, arch the back of the tongue toward the soft palate and bring the lips in, to a slightly rounded position.

Repeat the following aloud ten times:

ounce, our, out, owlish, cloud, bower, cower, doubt, down

flower, foul, house, mouse, mouth, proud, rout, south, towel

allow, avow, brow, chow, endow, plow, pow-wow, scow, vow

1. The clouds drifted above the plowed ground before the howling shower came.
2. Mrs. Brown found a mouse in the house.
3. The prow of the scow destroyed the cowing flowers.
4. The owlish clown has a proud brow and a foul mouth.

The U Family

u, As in Union

How to Produce Long *u*: Long *u* requires movement of tongue and lips. With lips relaxed and slightly spread, place the tip of the tongue behind the lower front teeth and arch the front of the tongue toward the front of the roof of the mouth. Press the sides of the tongue against the upper jaw teeth, as for *e* in eat. With a murmur, begin with the sound of long *e,* then arch the back of the tongue toward the soft palate while rounding and protruding the lips and making the *oo* sound for ooze.

Drill exercise:

e,e,e,   oo,oo,oo,   e,e,e,   oo,oo,oo,   e,e,e,   oo,oo,oo

e,oo,   e,oo,   e,oo,   e,oo,   e,oo,   e,oo   e,oo

Blend the two:

eoo,   eoo,   eoo,   eoo,   eoo,   eoo,   eoo,   eoo

u,u,u,   u,u,u,   u,u,u,   u,u,u,   u,u,u

Repeat the following aloud ten times:

cumulus, cucumber, cue, cumulate, cupid, bubonic, beautician

beautiful, cute, cuticle, dew, dune, fuel, bugle, plume, fume

Hubert, hue, huge, human, humor, music, musical, mutual, new

1. Bugles played as plumes of cumulus clouds accumulated over the dunes.

2. Beautiful music was heard over the hue created by Hubert's humor.

3. The musical humorist entitled his humorous composition "Humoresque."

4. Beulah was a beautiful cute baby with dewy eyes.

u, As in Up

How to Produce *u* As in Up: Place the tip of the tongue behind the lower front teeth, and raise the middle of the tongue slightly toward the roof of the mouth while expelling the breath with a grunt.

Repeat the following aloud ten times:

ugly, onion, other, oven, ulcer, ultimate, ultra, umpire, under

up, upward, us, usher, utter, utterance, bud, bug, chug, cuff

cup, dull, gulf, gull, hunt, judge, rough, run, skull, tough

1. Put the onion in the oven and the bug on the rug.
2. The ugly mutt was judged on the shape of his rough skull.

3. The utterance of the usher stunned the umpire under the tower.

4. The gulls hunted on the gulf while the mut dug in the rough mud.

The Short-Short U Family

a, As in Ago

For our purpose we shall coin a phrase: the *short-short u*. The short-short *u* sound is a neutral vowel, officially called *schwa*, (pronounced *shwa* and rhymes with *shah*.) The phonetic symbol for *schwa* or *short-short u*, is the upside-down *e* you find in the Pronunciation Key in your dictionary. This neutral vowel represents the following sounds: *a* in *ago*, *e* in *agent*, *i* in *sanity*, *o* in *comply*, and *u* in *focus*.

How to Produce the *short-short u*: Place the tip of the tongue behind the lower front teeth, and raise the middle of the tongue slightly toward the roof of the mouth, as for *u* in *up*. Now, expel the breath in a low short grunt.

Repeat the following aloud ten times:

ago, above, abandon, about, across, adore, affect, around, economy

equivalent, immature, impeccable, arena, pizza, Austria, Australia

bacteria, barracuda, cinema, data, pneumonia, Riviera

1. We shall not accuse and abuse the mischievous girl.
2. The occasion in Australia accidentally advanced the economy.
3. Lena was advised to abandon the pizza before she came across the abyss.
4. Rebecca looked about, above, and across and affected a mischievous air.

Chapter 4

CONSONANT COMBINATIONS
AT THE BEGINNING OF WORDS

There are 25 consonant combinations at the beginning of words. They are easily learned after the basic consonant sounds have been mastered. While *practicing* the combinations there are four things to keep in mind:

1. Overemphasize the consonant sounds.
2. Give only the sound, not the letter.
3. Drill on each sound separately, then combine the two.
4. Then, blend the two sounds so rapidly that they emerge as one sound.

The Bl Combination

Turn back and review the *b* and *l* sounds.

Drill exercise:

b,b,b,   l,l,l,   b,b,b,   l,l,l,   b,b,b,   l,l,l

b,l,   b,l,   b,l,   b,l,   b,l,   b,l,   b,l

bl,   bl,   bl,   bl,   bl,   bl,   bl,   bl

Repeat aloud the following ten times:

blue, black, blade, blight, blouse, bloom, blissful, blinker, blend

1. Blanch blew the blade of grass from the blackberries.
2. The blue blouse was bleached in the blustery wind.
3. The blazing blinkers blinded the driver.

4. The blast blew the blaze a block away.

5. Blueberries bloom blithely beside the door.

The Fl Combination

Review the *f* and *l* sounds.

Drill exercise:

f,f,f,   l,l,l,   f,f,f,   l,l,l,   f,f,f,   l,l,l

f,l,   f,l,   f,l,   f,l,   f,l,   f,l,   f,l

fl,   fl,   fl,   fl,   fl,   fl,   fl,   fl

Repeat the following aloud ten times:

flag, flame, flash, flee, flock, flea, flatter, flavor, flexible

1. Flocks of geese flashed across the sky fleeing wintry snowflakes.

2. Flora was a flapper in the Flaming Forties.

3. Flipper flung water at the people who flattered him.

4. Fluctuating flames flew up the chimney.

5. A flurry of flouncing skirts announced the beginning of the flamenco dance.

The Gl Combination

Review the *g* and *l* sounds.

Drill exercise:

g,g,g,   l,l,l,   g,g,g,   l,l,l,   g,g,g,   l,l,l

g,l,   g,l,   g,l,   g,l,   g,l,   g,l,   g,l

gl,   gl,   gl,   gl,   gl,   gl,   gl,   gl,

Repeat aloud the following ten times:

glide, glance, glare, glue, glen, gloom, glory, glimmer, glacier

1. The glimmer of the sunset dispelled the gloom in the glen.

2. The glow from the glass produced a glaze throughout the room.

3. Gloria glided across the room despite the glances of jealous girls.

The Cl (Kl) Combination

Review the *k* and *l* sounds.

Drill exercise:

k,k,k, l,l,l, k,k,k, l,l,l, k,k,k, l,l,l

k,l, k,l, k,l, k,l, k,l, k,l, k,l

kl, kl, kl, kl, kl, kl, kl, kl

Repeat the following aloud ten times:

clear, clad, clan, cloud, claim, cling, climate, classics, clasp

1. Cleavage between the generations caused a clash of personalities.

2. Clara received a clue to cleaning the clasp of her broach.

3. The cloistered clouds cleared the horizon in the summer climate.

4. Clean the clods from the climbing vine and claim the reward.

The Pl Combination

Review the *p* and *l* sounds.

Drill exercise:

p,p,p, l,l,l, p,p,p, l,l,l, p,p,p, l,l,l

p,l,　p,l,　p,l,　p,l,　p,l,　p,l,　p,l

pl,　pl,　pl,　pl,　pl,　pl,　pl,　pl

Repeat the following aloud ten times:

plume, place, plural, plow, plus, plump, plain, plank, pledge

1. The plate was placed on a plain plaid cloth.
2. Planks in his platform became a plucky pledge.
3. The playful platoon plundered the plum pudding.
4. Please plant plain tulips in a place beside the placid stream.

The Sl Combination

Review the *s* and *l* sounds.

Drill exercise:

s,s,s,　l,l,l,　s,s,s,　l,l,l,　s,s,s,　l,l,l

s,l,　s,l,　s,l,　s,l,　s,l,　s,l,　s,l

sl,　sl,　sl,　sl,　sl,　sl,　sl,　sl

Repeat the following ten times:

sleek, sly, sleep, sleeve, slang, slash, slant, sleigh, slothful

1. The slow, slothful boy sloshed through sleet and snow.
2. The snake slithered through the slushy and slimy sloop.
3. The oil slick became slimmer as he slipped the slurry into the water.
4. Sleigh bells were ringing as we slumbered in the sleet.

The Br Combination

Review the *b* and *r* sounds.

Drill exercise:

b,b,b,   r,r,r,   b,b,b,   r,r,r,   b,b,b,   r,r,r

b,r,   b,r,   b,r,   b,r,   b,r,   b,r,   b,r

br,   br,   br,   br,   br,   br,   br,   b,r

Repeat the following aloud ten times:

brain, brag, brand, brawl, breach, bright, broke, brilliant

1. The brilliant student broke the record for the broad jump.
2. He brought the broom to use for a brief unbroken moment.
2. The brush was brilliant in the sun.
4. Mr. Brown's brother brought a brief case to the brier patch.

The Dr Combination

Review the *d* and *r* sounds.

Drill exercise:

d,d,d,   r,r,r,   d,d,d,   r,r,r,   d,d,d,   r,r,r

d,r,   d,r,   d,r,   d,r,   d,r,   d,r,   d,r,

dr,   dr,   dr,   dr,   dr,   dr,   dr,   dr

Repeat the following aloud ten times:

drab, drain, drama, drink, draw, dream, dragon, driven, droll, driveway

1. We drove into the driveway as the drizzle set in.
2. The drooping dog dropped behind, drooling for his dinner.

3. High school dropouts frequently turn to drugs.

4. He drew water from the drinking fountain at the drawbridge.

The Fr Combination

Review the *f* and *r* sounds.

Drill exercise:

f,f,f,   r,r,r,   f,f,f,   r,r,r,   f,f,f,   r,r,r

f,r,   f,r,   f,r,   f,r,   f,r,   f,r,   f,r

fr,   fr,   fr,   fr,   fr,   fr,   fr,   fr

Repeat the following aloud ten times:

fresh, free, frank, frame, fraud, freak, freight, freeze, friend

1. Friends frequently frown at freshmen who get fresh.

2. Fred's frivolous friend frittered her time away.

3. Frontiersmen made a frontal attack against the enemy.

4. Freeloaders frequently fail.

The Gr Combination (Hard g)

Review the *g* and *r* sounds.

Drill exercise:

g,g,g,   r,r,r,   g,g,g,   r,r,r,   g,g,g,   r,r,r

g,r,   g,r,   g,r,   g,r,   g,r,   g,r,   g,r

gr,   gr,   gr,   gr,   gr,   gr,   gr,   gr

Repeat the following aloud ten times:

grain, grab, gravity, great, grub, graceful, graft, graph, grape

1. Greta became groggy with too much groovy music.

2. The Gross National Product was greatly overrated.

3. Ground-to-air missiles were grouped in a grotesque manner.

4. Grumpy players grumbled about the grime on the gridiron.

The Cr, Chr, and Kr Combination

Review the *k* and *r* sounds.

Drill exercise:

k,k,k,   r,r,r,   k,k,k,   r,r,r,   k,k,k,   r,r,r

k,r,   k,r,   k,r,   k,r,   k,r,   k,r,   k,r

kr,   kr,   kr,   kr,   kr,   kr,   kr,   kr

Repeat the following aloud ten times:

cry, crouch, cross, cream, Creole, cracker, crisp, crinkle, cram

1. The chrome on his Chrysler had corroded.

2. Christians meet crises without cringing.

3. Students are criticized for cramming at critical times.

4. Cruel crows crustily destroyed the farmer's crops.

The Pr Combination

Review the *p* and *r* sounds.

Drill exercise:

p,p,p,   r,r,r,   p,p,p,   r,r,r,   p,p,p,   r,r,r

p,r,   p,r,   p,r,   p,r,   p,r,   p,r,   p,r

pr,   pr,   pr,   pr,   pr,   pr,   pr,   pr

Repeat the following aloud ten times:

praise, prank, preserve, prepare, pride, prestige, prize, price

1. We presumed that the press preferred to print the truth.
2. His prestige was preserved through private practice.
3. Pretending to preserve the status quo, he prescribed drastic measures.
4. Those present were presented with presentable presents.

The Shr Combination

Review the *sh* and *r* sounds.

Drill exercise:

sh,sh,sh,   r,r,r,   sh,sh,sh,   r,r,r,   sh,sh,sh,   r,r,r

sh,r,   sh,r,   sh,r,   sh,r,   sh,r,   sh,r,   sh,r

shr,   shr,   shr,   shr,   shr,   shr,   shr,   shr

Repeat the following aloud ten times:

shrink, shrapnal, shrivel, shrine, shrewd, shrill, shrub, shrug

1. We heard the shrill whistle of shrimp boats as they shrank from view.
2. The shrieking of laughter should never be heard near a religious shrine.
3. Shrewd merchants do not allow for shrinkage.
4. Shrewd students never shrug off new ideas.

The Thr Combination (Th As in They)

Review the *th* and *r* sounds.

Drill exercise:

th,th,th,   r,r,r,   th,th,th,   r,r,r,   th,th,th,   r,r,r

th,r,   th,r,   th,r,   th,r,   th,r,   th,r,   th,r

thr,   thr,   thr,   thr,   thr,   thr,   thr,   thr

Repeat the following aloud ten times:

thrash, threshold, thread, threat, thrift, thrill, throb, thrive

1. The throbbing of the thrasher means that thrifty men are thriving.

2. The engine gave a throaty throb as it was thrown in reverse.

3. Three brown thrashers threatened to thrash the jay-bird.

5. She was thrilled when she began to thrive from thrifty business deals.

The Tr Combination

Review the *t* and *r* sounds

Drill exercise:

t,t,t,   r,r,r,   t,t,t,   r,r,r,   t,t,t,   r,r,r

t,r,   t,r,   t,r,   t,r,   t,r,   t,r,   t,r

tr,   tr,   tr,   tr,   tr,   tr,   tr,   tr

Repeat the following aloud ten times:

track, trade, trace, trail, trait, trample, tread, try, trap

1. Smoke trails traced the trawler as it traveled through the dusk.

2. The boy was trapped in the trailer when he trans-ferred the trampoline.

3. The trail boss trounced the traitor for trying to make trouble.

4. It is tragic to try and fail when trying harder would succeed.

The Qu (Kw) Combination

Review the *k* and *w* sounds.

Drill exercise:

k,k,k,   w,w,w,   k,k,k,   w,w,w,   k,k,k,   w,w,w

k,w,   k,w,   k,w,   k,w,   k,w,   k,w,   k,w

kw,   kw,   kw,   kw,   kw,   kw,   kw,   kw

Repeat the following aloud ten times:

quack, quail, quantity, quality, quandary, quarantine, quarrel

1. The quantity of the quartz will depend on its quality.

2. The queen developed a queasy feeling after eating too quickly.

3. The queer-looking quill elicited a quip from the quintuplets.

4. The quartet quietly quarreled about the quaver in their voices.

The Sw Combination

Review the *s* and *w* sounds.

Drill exercise:

s,s,s,   w,w,w,   s,s,s,   w,w,w,   s,s,s,   w,w,w

s,w,   s,w,   s,w,   s,w,   s,w,   s,w,   s,w

sw,   sw,,   sw,   sw,   sw,   sw,   sw,   sw

Repeat the following aloud ten times:

swab, swag, swim, swear, sweat, sweep, sweet, swarm, sway

1. The sailor swaggered on board and began swabbing the deck.

2. Swallows swing effortlessly above the swimmers.

3. A short, swarthy man swept the swallowtail onto the sward.

4. The swiftly flying swan sweltered in the sweeping sunrays.

The Tw Combination

Review the *t* and *w* sounds.

Drill exercise:

t,t,t,   w,w,w,   t,t,t,   w,w,w,   t,t,t,   w,w,w

t,w,   t,w,   t,w,   t,w,   t,w,   t,w,   t,w

tw,   tw,   tw,   tw,   tw,   tw,   tw,   tw

Repeat the following aloud ten times:

twaddle, twang, tweed, twig, twiddle, twin, twinkle, tweezers, tweak

1. If a twig were twins, twelve twigs would equal twenty-four.

2. Tweezers were used to tweak the ears of the twaddling girls.

3. Tweedledee and Tweedledum twiddled through their twangy duet.

4. Twilight comes twice in a twenty-four hour day.

The Sf (Sph) Combination

Review the *s* and *f* sounds. Ph has the sound of f.

Drill exercise:

> s,s,s, f,f,f, s,s,s, f,f,f, s,s,s, f,f,f
>
> s,f, s,f, s,f, s,f, s,f, s,f, s,f
>
> sf, sf, sf, sf, sf, sf, sf, sf

Repeat the following aloud ten times:

> sphere, sphagnum, sphinx, spherical, spheroid, sphenoid, sphene

1. The sphinx of ancient Egypt was an imaginary creature.

2. The earth is spherical in shape.

3. Does the western hemisphere include both the United States and Russia?

The Sk (Sc, Sch, Squ) Combination

Review the *s* and *k* sounds.

Drill exercise:

> s,s,s, k,k,k, s,s,s, k,k,k, s,s,s, k,k,k
>
> s,k, s,k, s,k, s,k, s,k, s,k, s,k
>
> sk, sk, sk, sk, sk, sk, sk, sk

Repeat the following aloud ten times:

> scare, scold, scald, scallop, scamp, squall, scarves, scheme, school

1. The screeching of brakes near the school resulted in a scathing scolding.

2. The sceptics scoffed at the claim of feminine screams at the schoolhouse.

3. The scathing remarks scotched the scamp's attempt to scrawl on the wall.

4. The scope of the scheme scared the participants away.

The Sn Combination

Review the *s* and *n* sounds.

Drill exercise:

s,s,s,   n,n,n,   s,s,s,   n,n,n,   s,s,s,   n,n,n

s,n,   s,n,   s,n,   s,n,   s,n,   s,n,   s,n

sn,   sn,   sn,   sn,   sn,   sn,   sn,   sn

Repeat the following aloud ten times:

snag, snail, snake, snap, snare, sneer, snob, snub, snow, snarl

1. The student snored loudly while he snoozed in the classroom.

2. He gave a snide remark about the sneers and snickers he encountered.

3. The sniveling sniper snitched on the snob who snubbed the woman.

4. Snipes, snails, and snakes caused the boy to sneeze.

The Sm Combination

Review the *s* and *m* sounds.

Drill exercise:

s,s,s,   m,m,m,   s,s,s,   m,m,m,   s,s,s,   m,m,m

s,m,   s,m,   s,m,   s,m,   s,m,   s,m,   s,m

sm,   sm,   sm,   sm,   sm,   sm,   sm,   sm

Repeat the following aloud ten times:

small, smart, smear, smile, smirk, smirch, smoke, smooth, smug

1. Smart girls wear smocks to guard against smudges.
2. Smutty smoke smouldered above the smudge pots.
3. Smoke-eaters smoothly smothered the smouldering flames.
4. The small, smart boy smugly smashed the smutty window.

The Sp Combination

Review the *s* and *p* sounds.

Drill exercise:

s,s,s, p,p,p, s,s,s, p,p,p, s,s,s, p,p,p

s,p, s,p, s,p, s,p, s,p, s,p, s,p

sp, sp, sp, sp, sp, sp, sp, sp

Repeat the following aloud ten times:

space, spade, span, speech, speak, spice, speck, spend, speed

1. The spirit of the space age is spanning the world.
2. A spanking breeze brought the smell of spices.
3. The speaker held us spellbound with his spiel for spending less.
4. Water sprites spent a moment spatting before speeding away on spindly legs.

The St Combination

Review the *s* and *t* sounds.

Drill exercise:

s,s,s, t,t,t, s,s,s, t,t,t, s,s,s, t,t,t

s,t,   *s,t,*   *s,t,*   *s,t,*   *s,t,*   *s,t,*   *sf,t*

st,   *st,*   *st,*   *st,*   *st,*   *st,*   *st,*   *st*

Repeat the following aloud ten times:

stare, state, stain, stale, staple, stable, star, stair, stamp

1. He staked his reputation on building a stairway to the stars.

2. The sponsor used a spade to dislodge the spong.

3. In spring the sprigs became spotted with spreading spores.

4. Staple crops remained stable and were stored by a state staff.

The Wh Combination

Review the *w* and *h* sounds.

Drill exercise:

w,w,w,   *h,h,h,*   *w,w,w,*   *h,h,h,*   *w,w,w,*   *h,h,h*

w,h,   *w,h,*   *w,h,*   *w,h,*   *w,h,*   *w,h,*   *w,h*

wh,   *wh,*   *wh,*   *wh,*   *wh,*   *wh,*   *wh,*   *wh*

Repeat the following aloud ten times:

whack, white, whale, wharf, wheat, wheel, when, whether, whimper

1. Why must we whitewash what we do wrong?

2. The whistler waited a while under the whispering gallery.

3. He whetted the whetstone where white water whispered.

4. The whorls on the wheel seemed to whirl.

Chapter 5

SOME TROUBLESOME ENDINGS

Words Ending in *ed*

The final *ed* is pronounced *d* in some words, but *t* in others. For example, *begged* is pronounced (begd); but baked is pronounced (bakt.) When *ed* represents the past tense or past participle of a verb, *without forming an extra syllable,* it is pronounced *d,* IF the preceding sound is a *voiced* sound, as in the following words.

The Final D Sound

Repeat the following aloud ten times, exaggerating the *d* sound:

beg, begged   care, cared

rub, rubbed   pull, pulled

bathe, bathed   flow, flowed

charge, charged   will, willed

scream, screamed   play, played

ooz, oozed   clean, cleaned

gain, gained   call, called

1. He begged to have his back rubbed while he bathed.
2. The woman screamed for being charged when she gained a profit.

3. The creamed pie flowed from the box when it oozed out.

4. She called to say that she cared.

5. He pulled the furniture out and cleaned the room.

The Final T Sound

When final *ed* represents the past tense or past participle of a verb, without forming an extra syllable, it is pronounced *t,* if the preceding sound is a *voiceless* or *whispered* sound.

Repeat the following aloud ten times, exaggerating the *t* sound:

bake, baked   wrap, wrapped

reach, reached   pass, passed

laugh, laughed   rush, rushed

match, matched   cough, coughed

ask, asked   milk, milked

bless, blessed (verb)   crook, crooked (verb)

spank, spanked   help, helped

1. She baked a cake yesterday.

2. He passed and said that he had reached a decision.

3. The wrapped scarves matched perfectly.

4. I shall ask him now because you asked him yesterday.

5. She coughed and asked to be helped to her seat.

Words Ending in s, es, and 's
The z Sound

When words ending in *s, es, and 's* indicate the plural or possessive forms of nouns or the third person singular form of verbs, the final sound is pronounced *z* when the preceding sound is a *voiced* sound.

Repeat the following ten times, exaggerating the *z* sound:

goes, rubs, comes, dogs, gives, birds, sins, sings, cars, halls

Fred's barns, dabbles, ruffles, giggles, baths, chasms, schisms

1. The girls' giggles disturbed the birds taking baths.
2. Fred's dogs avoided many chasms while hunting.
3. Hogs were kept in barns on Carl's farm.
4. He robs the birds and gives the eggs away.
5. Here comes the boy who sells bottles, and prattles about schisms.

The s Sound

When words ending in *s, es, and 's* indicate the plural or possessive forms of nouns or the third person singular form of verbs, the final sound is pronounced *s* when the preceding sound is a *voiceless,* or *whispered* sound.

Repeat the following aloud ten times, exaggerating the *s* sound:

caps, hats, docks, fifes, backs, coughs, laughs, drifts

asks, spanks, calms, healths, months, harps, milks, helps

1. She laughs as she wraps paper around the harps.
2. Their coughs lasted many months.
3. Caps and hats were doffed when the fifes began to play.
4. He helps when she milks the cows.
5. Drifts of snow lasted many months.

EDIT YOURSELF

Edit Yourself

A Manual For Everyone
Who Works With Words

by BRUCE ROSS-LARSON

W·W·NORTON & COMPANY   New York   London

LIBRARY OF CONGRESS CATALOGING IN PUBLICATION DATA

Ross-Larson, Bruce Clifford, 1942–
  Edit yourself.

  1. English language—Rhetoric. 2. English
language—Grammar—1950-   . 3. Authorship—
Handbooks, manuals, etc. 4. Editing. I. Title.
PE1408.R725 1982   808'.042   82-6432
                                    AACR2

ISBN 0-393-01640-4

W. W. Norton & Company, Inc. 500 Fifth Avenue, New York, N.Y. 10110
W. W. Norton & Company Ltd. 37 Great Russell Street, London WC1B 3NU

  2 3 4 5 6 7 8 9 0

TO GODDARD WINTERBOTTOM
for showing the way

Contents

Author's Note

In the first part of this book I have drawn together solutions to the more common problems of everyday writing, such problems as fat, inconsistency, and the failure to use parallel grammatical constructions. In the second part I have arranged, in alphabetical order, more than fifteen hundred common cuts, changes, and comparisons that editors make to produce clear, concise writing. The recommendations in that part enlarge on the solutions proposed in the first two chapters of part I: "Fat" and "The Better Word." Those recommendations would, I admit, reduce great prose to the ordinary. But if followed, they can lift ordinary writing to a plane of greater clarity and distinction.

Bruce Ross-Larson

Acknowledgments

For suggestions about the shape and content of this book and for guidance on many problems of editing, I owe much to Harriet Baldwin, Jane Carroll, Carl Dahlman, George Dorsey, David Driscoll, Richard Herbert, Virginia Hitchcock, Andrea Hodson, David Howell Jones, Starling Lawrence, James McEuen, Ricardo Moran, Marilyn Silverman, Brian Svikhart, Kim Tran, Larry Westphal, Goddard Winterbottom, and especially Edward Hodnett. I also owe much to the books I frequently pull from my shelf: *Webster's New Collegiate Dictionary*, Strunk and White's *Elements of Style*, Fowler's *Modern English Usage*, Follett's *Modern American Usage*, Gowers's *Complete Plain Words*, Flesch's *ABC of Style*, the University of Chicago Press's *Manual of Style*, and Prentice-Hall's *Handbook for Writers* and *Words into Type*.

Part I **WHAT EDITORS
LOOK FOR**

Chapter 1 **Fat**

Just as your speech is filled with many words that add nothing to what you say, your writing is often larded with words that obscure your meaning rather than clarify it. Trim this fat off to direct your reader's attention to important words and ideas.

SUPERFLUOUS NOUNS

Superfluous nouns fatten many sentences and distract attention from a stronger noun by relegating it to a prepositional phrase.

the field of economics	CHANGE TO	economics
the level of wages rose	CHANGE TO	wages rose
the process of indus- trialization	CHANGE TO	industrialization
the volume of demand fell	CHANGE TO	demand fell

Such trimming does not always work, but it does work often. Here is a list of nouns that, interposed between *the* and *of*, can often be done away with.

the amount of	CUT
the area of	CUT
the case of	CUT

the character of	CUT
the concept of	CUT
the degree of	CUT
the existence of	CUT
the extent of	CUT
the field of	CUT
the form of	CUT
the idea of	CUT
the level of	CUT
the magnitude of	CUT
the nature of	CUT
the number of	CUT
the presence of	CUT
the process of	CUT
the purpose of	CUT
the sum of	CUT
the volume of	CUT
the way of	CUT

SUPERFLUOUS VERBS

There are two classes of superfluous verb. One is an array of pretenders—idle, common verbs that supplant a working verb, which becomes a noun: such verbs as *do, have, make, provide,* and *serve.*

do a study of the effects	CHANGE TO	study the effects
have a tendency to	CHANGE TO	tend to
make changes in the	CHANGE TO	change the
make decisions about	CHANGE TO	decide on
make progress toward	CHANGE TO	progress toward
provide a summary of the	CHANGE TO	summarize the
serve to make reductions	CHANGE TO	reduce

This formula changes the objective noun to a verb and displaces the pretender. Take care, however, not to be too zealous in applying this formula, or you will end up with such artificial verbs as *prioritize,* from *priority.*

The second class of superfluous verb is found in a clause that modifies a noun. Such verbs, along with the pronouns and helping verbs that precede them, can often be deleted.

the ice that is contained in	CHANGE TO	the ice in
the people who are concerned are	CHANGE TO	the people are
the argument that is included in the	CHANGE TO	the argument in
the tasks that are involved in	CHANGE TO	the tasks in
the people who are located in	CHANGE TO	the people in
the numbers shown in the	CHANGE TO	the numbers in the
the estimates presented in the	CHANGE TO	the estimates in the
the facts given in the	CHANGE TO	the facts in the

SUPERFLUOUS ARTICLES AND PREPOSITIONS

the making of cloth	CHANGE TO	making cloth
the manufacture of steel	CHANGE TO	manufacturing steel
many of the countries	CHANGE TO	many countries
several of the countries	CHANGE TO	several countries
some of the countries	CHANGE TO	some countries
fill up the tank	CHANGE TO	fill the tank
lay out the pipes	CHANGE TO	lay the pipes

Note that these recommendations can sometimes change the meaning. If they do, let the original construction stand.

THE OPENING "IT"

Two classes of the opening *It* indicate fat. The first is *It is . . .* , *It was . . .* , or *It will be . . .* , followed by the subject, followed by *who*, *that*, or *which*. The construction sometimes is justifiable for emphasis, but it generally is unacceptable because it gives the prominent lead position in the sentence to a pronoun not yet defined, a position that the subject deserves. It takes, in addition, three more words.

It is Richard who damaged . . .	CHANGE TO	Richard damaged . . .

| It was Wang Laboratories that engineered . . . | CHANGE TO | Wang Laboratories engineered . . . |

The second class is a series of circumlocutions—of uses of many words where fewer will do—that begin with the indefinite pronoun *It*.

It appears that Cuba will . . .	CHANGE TO	Cuba will . . .
It goes without saying that I . . .	CHANGE TO	I . . .
It should be noted that I . . .	CHANGE TO	I . . .

Almost any sentence will be improved by trimming such fatty constructions.

THE OPENING "THERE"

Two classes of the opening *There* should be avoided. The first is the same as the first class of the opening *It*.

| There are some buildings that will . . . | CHANGE TO | Some buildings will . . . |
| There are some people who are . . . | CHANGE TO | Some people are . . . |

The second class relegates what might precede the verb to less prominence after the verb.

| There is nothing wrong with the opening *there*, unless there are too many *there*'s in evidence. | CHANGE TO | Nothing is wrong with the opening *there*, unless too many *there*'s are evident. |

Note that such rescues are not always felicitous: *There are two reasons* should not be changed to *Reasons are two*.

OVERWEIGHT PREPOSITIONS

Many overweight phrases needlessly detract from the objects they introduce by fattening a sentence. Here are some samples of phrases that should usually be replaced by shorter prepositions.

as regards	CHANGE TO	on, for, about
as to	CUT OR CHANGE TO	in, of, on, for, about
concerning	CHANGE TO	at, of, on, for, about
in regard to	CHANGE TO	on, about
in relation to	CHANGE TO	on, about
in respect to	CHANGE TO	on, about
in terms of	TRY	as, at, by, in, of, for, with, under, through
regarding	TRY	on, for, about
related to	TRY	of, on, about
relating to	TRY	on, for, about
with reference to	CHANGE TO	of, on, for, about
with respect to	CHANGE TO	on, for, about

WEAKLING MODIFIERS

Weakling modifiers, permissible perhaps once in a manuscript for emphasis, can almost always be removed without changing the meaning of a sentence.

active	CUT
actively	CUT
actual	CUT
actually	CUT
any	CUT
available	CUT
both	CUT
careful	CUT
carefully	CUT
certain	CUT
certainly	CUT
comparative	CUT
comparatively	CUT
definite	CUT
definitely	CUT
effective	CUT
eminent	CUT
eminently	CUT
existing	CUT
fortunately	CUT
herself	CUT
himself	CUT
hopefully	CUT

in fact	CUT
in general	CUT
in particular	CUT
in the future	CUT
in the past	CUT
indeed	CUT
inevitably	CUT
itself	CUT
meaningful	CUT
meaningfully	CUT
namely	CUT
necessarily	CUT
needless to say	CUT
now	CUT
over time	CUT
overall	CUT
particular	CUT
particularly	CUT
per se	CUT
pretty	CUT
quite	CUT
rather	CUT
real	CUT
really	CUT
relative	CUT
relatively	CUT
respective	CUT
respectively	CUT
somewhat	CUT
specific	CUT
themselves	CUT
total	CUT
unfortunately	CUT
very	CUT

See the alphabetized entries in part II for more fat that can be trimmed off your sentences.

Chapter 2 The Better Word

Some words are better than others because they are correct, because they are right for the audience, because they illuminate an idea for the reader, or because they are preferred by most good writers most of the time. The more often you use the better word, the better your writing will seem to others.

Because there are so many possibilities, only a few examples are given under each heading to indicate what to be on the lookout for. Note that many problems can be avoided simply by referring to the dictionary, which should be at hand when you are writing or editing.

WHAT TO PREFER

Prefer short words to long

accomplish	CHANGE TO	do
component	CHANGE TO	part
facilitate	TRY	ease, help, make easier
lengthy	CHANGE TO	long
utilization	TRY	use

Prefer concrete words to abstract

One red flag for abstraction is the suffix *-ion*. A subject ending in *-ion* should be scrutinized to see whether it can be replaced by a concrete word.

9

diction	CHANGE TO	choice of words
prestidigitation	TRY	sleight of hand
variation in skill	TRY	different ability

Prefer specific words to general

facility	TRY	office building
lower-tract discomfort	TRY	diarrhea
natural fertilizer	TRY	cow dung
several	TRY	six
vehicle	TRY	car

Prefer everyday language to jargon

If jargon must be used, it should be defined in parentheses on its first appearance.

adult literacy rate	TRY	percentage of people over fifteen who can read and write
five megabyte	TRY	five million characters
morbidity and mortality	TRY	illness and death

Prefer singular nouns to plural

The distinction depends on whether you are writing about what makes up the aggregate or about the aggregate. If the second, use the singular and see how your writing improves.

benefits	CHANGE TO	benefit
costs	CHANGE TO	cost
elites	CHANGE TO	elite
expenditures	CHANGE TO	expenditure
moneys	CHANGE TO	money
pressures	CHANGE TO	pressure
revenues	CHANGE TO	revenue

See part II of this book for more plural nouns that can often be singular.

Prefer words to symbols, initials, and abbreviations

If symbols, initials, and abbreviations must be used, they should be defined on their first appearance: for example, the gross national product (GNP).

etc.	CHANGE TO	and so on, and so forth
e.g.	CHANGE TO	for example
km.	CHANGE TO	kilometers
%	CHANGE TO	percent
CDR	CHANGE TO	the crude death rate

Prefer American words and phrases to foreign

Foreign words and phrases include British idiosyncrasies *(as regards)*. Recommendations for the treatment of Latin words, phrases, and abbreviations are drawn together at the end of part II.

a priori	TRY	deductive(ly), presumptive(ly)
as regards	CHANGE TO	on, for, about
ceteris paribus	CHANGE TO	other things being equal

Prefer familiar words to unfamiliar

defalcate	CHANGE TO	embezzle
defenestrate	CHANGE TO	throw out of a window
shrewdness of gorillas	CHANGE TO	family of gorillas

WHAT TO AVOID

Avoid contractions

| don't | CHANGE TO | do not |
| here's | CHANGE TO | here is |

Avoid ugly words ending in -wise and -ize

A few uses of the suffix *-wise* are legitimate: *clockwise, likewise, lengthwise,* and *otherwise.* Other uses border on excess, as do many uses of the suffix *-ize.*

| electricitywise | CHANGE TO | about electricity |
| prioritize | CHANGE TO | set priorities for |

Avoid overused phrases (and fad words and slang)

impact [as a verb]	CHANGE TO	affect, have an effect
interface	TRY	work together
bottom line	CHANGE TO	what this means
rationale	TRY	reason

WHAT ELSE TO WATCH

Watch prepositions

Many dictionaries, in their examples of usage, offer help on preferred prepositions. Part II of this book also has solutions to some of
the more common mistakes.

conform with	CHANGE TO	conform to
correspond with [by letter]	COMPARE	correspond to [match, go with]
integrate into	CHANGE TO	integrate with
investigation into	CHANGE TO	investigation of

Watch seeming synonyms

There are two opposing tendencies in American usage. One is to
attach one meaning to many words, making them synonyms. The
other is to reserve one meaning for one word, another for another,
keeping them distinct. The first tendency is a lapse into sloth, the
second a desire for precision. Part II of this book gives more exten-
sive advice on some of the more troublesome pairs and threesomes.

among [three or more]	COMPARE	between [two or two at a time]
contemptible [deserving scorn]	COMPARE	contemptuous [scornful]
imply [suggest]	COMPARE	infer [conclude]
masterful [strong-willed]	COMPARE	masterly [skillful]

Chapter 3   Pronoun References

Few things slow a reader down more than unclear pronoun references—signs of carelessness that quickly distract the reader from your meaning. The reader can usually divine what you mean, but only at a cost that need not be incurred. Here are two examples of the problem.

> *The main problem that people run into with pronouns arises*
> *from their . . .*

Does *their* refer to *people* or *pronouns?* The unfolding of the sentence may or may not give the answer.

> *The main problem that people run into with a pronoun is not*
> *tying it to its noun. It . . .*

Does *it* refer to *problem, pronoun, not tying it,* or *its noun?* Or is *it* indefinite? Again, the unfolding of the sentence may or may not give the answer.

That is why you should check each pronoun, whether personal, impersonal, relative, possessive, or substantive, to be sure that there is no question about the nouns that pronouns stand for.

AMBIGUOUS PRONOUNS

If two or three nouns vie for a pronoun, the reference is almost certain to be ambiguous. The general solutions are to repeat the noun rather than use a pronoun or to eliminate the pretenders by changing their number.

The main problems that people run into with pronouns arise from their not being tied to a noun.	CHANGE TO	The main problems that people run into with pronouns arise from a pronoun's not being tied to a noun.
	OR	The main problem that a writer has with pronouns arises from their not being tied to a noun.
Reagan told Haig that he would not serve a second term.	CHANGE TO	Reagan told Haig that he, Reagan, would not serve a second term.

DISTANT PRONOUNS

Another big problem with pronouns is introducing them at some distance from their noun. That sets the pronoun adrift. It is solved by repeating the noun that the distant pronoun stands for.	CHANGE TO	Another big problem with pronouns is introducing them at some distance from their noun. That sets the pronoun adrift. The problem is solved by repeating the noun that the distant pronoun stands for.

PREMATURE PRONOUNS

If it is unambiguously tied to the noun it stands for, a pronoun . . .	CHANGE TO	If a pronoun is unambiguously tied to the noun it stands for, it . . .
If she wins an Oscar for her performance, Meryl Streep will be the . . .	CHANGE TO	If Meryl Streep wins an Oscar for her performance, she will be the . . .

VAGUE PRONOUNS

If *this, that, these,* and *those* are used not as adjectives, as in *This book is* . . . , but as pronouns, as in *This is* . . . , they often are vague. If there is any question, however fleeting, about what the pronoun refers to, restore the noun or create one.

Several countries have objected to recent decisions by the U.S. government to deplete its stockpile of tin. These will lodge a . . .	CHANGE TO	Several countries have objected to recent decisions by the U.S. government to deplete its stockpile of tin. These countries will lodge a . . .
The White House proposed an increase in aid to El Salvador. This has set off a barrage . . .	CHANGE TO	The White House proposed an increase in aid to El Salvador. This proposal has set off a barrage of . . .

Note that such pronouns can stand alone if a verb separates them from what they stand for: *This is the reason that* . . . ; *These are times that.* . . .

ILLOGICAL PRONOUNS

Some pronouns illogically stand for a noun that is implicit, not stated.

Japan's exports of cars skyrocketed in the 1970s. The main reason is their skill in production.	CHANGE TO	Japan's exports of cars skyrocketed in the 1970s. The main reason is the skill of the Japanese in production.

Other pronouns illogically stand for nouns of a different number: that is, a singular pronoun stands for a plural noun, a plural pronoun for a singular noun.

Everyone has a right to the information they need to . . .	CHANGE TO	All people have a right to the information they need to . . .

	OR	Everyone has a right to the information he (or she) needs to . . .
Neither of the sloops have their crew aboard.	CHANGE TO	Neither of the sloops has its crew aboard.

Chapter 4 **Order in the Sentence**

The elements of pairs, series, and compound subjects and predicates usually appear as they come out of the writer's mind—haphazardly or alphabetically. Rearranging those elements from short to long, from simple to compound, increases the ability of the reader to understand them.

COUNT THE SYLLABLES

letters and arts	CHANGE TO	arts and letters
oranges and pears	CHANGE TO	pears and oranges

If the number of syllables is the same, count the letters.

COUNT THE WORDS

old-style politicians and reformers	CHANGE TO	reformers and old-style politicians
Raiders of the Lost Ark, Shane, and *Gone with the Wind*	CHANGE TO	*Shane, Gone with the Wind,* and *Raiders of the Lost Ark*
Romeo and Juliet, Macbeth, and *King Lear*	CHANGE TO	*Macbeth, King Lear,* and *Romeo and Juliet*
Washington, D.C., New York, and Miami	CHANGE TO	Miami, New York, and Washington, D.C.

17

PUT COMPOUND ELEMENTS LAST

liberty, the pursuit of happiness, and life	CHANGE TO	life, liberty, and the pursuit of happiness
He washed the glasses, dishes, and silverware, made the bed, and mopped the floor.	CHANGE TO	He made the bed, mopped the floor, and washed the dishes, glasses, and silverware.
The generally poor quality of education in public schools and crime are the main reasons.	CHANGE TO	Crime and the generally poor quality of education in public schools are the main reasons.
. . . from foreign suppliers of machinery, raw materials, and equipment or from foreign buyers.	CHANGE TO	. . . from foreign buyers or from foreign suppliers of equipment, machinery, and raw materials.

EXCEPTIONS

This simple way of injecting order into a disorderly sentence does not work all the time.

Obvious sequence or chronology

rites of life, birth, and death	CHANGE TO	rites of birth, life, and death
tea with lunch, dinner, and breakfast	CHANGE TO	tea with breakfast, lunch, and dinner

Unintended modifiers

the remarkable Divine and Tab Hunter	CHANGE TO	Tab Hunter and the remarkable Divine
trade and money-market rates	CHANGE TO	money-market rates and trade

Familiar or explicit order

cream and peaches	CHANGE TO	peaches and cream
the bees and the birds	CHANGE TO	the birds and the bees
gold, myrrh, and frankincense	CHANGE TO	gold, frankincense, and myrrh

Borg, Connors, and McEnroe were the three leading money-winners.

CHANGE TO

McEnroe, Borg, and Connors were the three leading money-winners, in that order.

Chapter 5 Shorter Sentences

Long sentences—those of more than, say, twenty words—often are hard to read. Short sentences usually are not. Successions of long sentences are even harder to read. But broken up by the occasional short sentence, successions of long sentences are easier to read.

So it is that the appeal of every writer on style is: Be brief! And so it is that the retort of every writer who lacks style is: It's not possible. Along with such corollaries as: Complicated ideas call for complicated sentences. Or: Short sentences lack style because they are choppy. The idea, however, is not to be brief all the time or even most of the time. The idea is to be brief unless you have a reason not to be. Even if you have a reason not to be brief, there are ways of handling a sentence that make it easier for your reader to follow what you are trying to say.

BREAK A LONG SENTENCE INTO TWO OR MORE SENTENCES

Kissinger, though paid $15,000 for an afternoon of talk, probably felt that the egg on his face was not worth it, and he must still be wondering how a person once all powerful could be sub-	CHANGE TO	Kissinger, though paid $15,000 for an afternoon of talk, probably felt that the egg on his face was not worth it. He must still be wondering how a person once all pow-

jected to such igno-
miny.

erful could be subjected
to such ignominy.

Even long sentences that read well can be broken down to add
emphasis or ease the task of the reader.

The immediate effects of the new economic policies have been to strike a bit of terror in the hearts of government workers, to plant smiles on the faces of the rich, and to put frowns on the faces of the poor, who have long benefited from the federal safety net.	TRY	The new economic policies have had three immediate effects. They have struck a bit of terror in the hearts of government workers. They have planted smiles on the faces of the rich. And they have put frowns on the faces of the poor, who have long benefited from the federal safety net.

CUT UNNECESSARY PHRASES AND CLAUSES

All subordinate clauses should be scrutinized to see if they con-
tribute to the thought. If not, they should be cut.

And they have put frowns on the faces of the poor, who have long benefited from the federal safety net.	CHANGE TO	And they have put frowns on the faces of the poor.
The problem, which remarkably few writers are aware of, is that of failing to set off a non-restrictive clause by punctuation—whether by commas, dashes, or parentheses.	CHANGE TO	The problem is that of failing to set off a non-restrictive clause by punctuation.

The same fate should befall the fat in a sentence.

The process of indus-trialization has served to help raise the GNP of many of the world's countries.	CHANGE TO	Industrialization has boosted the GNP of many countries.

JUDICIOUS REARRANGEMENT AND PUNCTUATION

Even if the length of a sentence stays much the same, judicious rearrangement and punctuation can give shape to otherwise amorphous elements.

Striking a bit of terror in the hearts of government workers, planting smiles on the faces of the rich, and putting frowns on the faces of the poor, who have long benefited from the federal safety net, have been the three immediate effects of the new economic policies.	TRY	The new economic policies have had three immediate effects: they have struck a bit of terror in the hearts of government workers, planted smiles on the faces of the rich, and put frowns on the faces of the poor people, who have long benefited from the federal safety net.

Dashes should occasionally be used to set off parenthetical material that separates a subject from its verb.

Long sentences, which can be defined as those of more than, say, twenty words, often are hard to read.	CHANGE TO	Long sentences—those of more than, say, twenty words—often are hard to read.

Chapter 6 **Dangling Constructions**

Danglers are easy to avoid, generally by moving what they refer to immediately after them. The only difficult thing about danglers is learning to recognize them.

PARTICIPLES

The most notorious dangler is the participle that introduces a phrase at the beginning of a sentence.

DANGLING		ATTACHED
Walking to work after the blizzard, the sun's reflection on the snow almost blinded him.	CHANGE TO	While walking to work after the blizzard, he was almost blinded by the sun's reflection on the snow.
	OR	While he was walking to work after the blizzard, the sun's reflection on the snow almost blinded him.
Using official data and other information, these costs were allocated to specific activities.	CHANGE TO	Using official data and other information, we allocated these costs to specific activities.

23

	OR	Official data and other information were used to allocate these costs to specific activities.
Transposing the elements of the main clause, the dangling clause was tied to the subject by the author.	CHANGE TO	By transposing the elements of the main clause, the author tied the dangling clause to the subject.

In the foregoing examples on the left, the dangling constructions have the following unfortunate effects on meaning: *the dangling clause* is *transposing the elements; these costs* are *using official data;* and *the sun's reflection* is *walking to work.*

OTHER PARTS

DANGLING		ATTACHED
Before applying to graduate school, it is a good idea to master dangling gerunds.	CHANGE TO	Before you apply to graduate school, you should master dangling gerunds.
Once in graduate school, it is wise to be on the lookout for dangling elliptical clauses.	CHANGE TO	Once in graduate school, you would be wise to be on the lookout for dangling elliptical clauses.
	OR	Once you are in graduate school, you would be wise to be on the lookout for dangling elliptical clauses.
To get into graduate school, it is necessary to have mastered dangling infinitives.	CHANGE TO	To get into graduate school, you must have mastered dangling infinitives.

The red flag for a dangler is a sentence with an introductory word, phrase, or clause. To recognize the problem, see whether the introductory matter applies to what immediately follows it. To solve the problem, transpose the elements of the main clause. Or rewrite either the main clause or the introductory matter to attach properly what would otherwise be unattached or incorrectly attached.

Chapter 7 **Abused Relatives**

That, which, and *who* are often used as relative pronouns to introduce clauses that modify the nouns they follow. They are three of the most useful, and used, words in the language. Being so useful, they often are misused or overused.

Two definitions are in order. A *restrictive clause*, which also is called a defining or limiting clause, defines a noun. A *nonrestrictive clause*, also called an informing or commenting clause, adds information about a noun that has already been defined or does not need definition. Here are some examples.

RESTRICTIVE CLAUSES	NONRESTRICTIVE CLAUSES
The book that (or which) I wrote in 1981 is about French politics.	My book on French politics, which I wrote in 1981, is about to be published.
The people who live next door are going to Hollywood.	The Moores, who live next door, are going to Hollywood.

A few comments should help clarify the differences between restrictive and nonrestrictive clauses even more. First, a restrictive clause can be introduced by *that, which*, or *who;* a nonrestrictive clause, by *which* or *who*. Second, in the foregoing examples of restrictive clauses, it is not known which *book* or which *people* are being written about until the clauses appears. The restrictive clause is needed to define

25

the *book* to distinguish it from other books and to define the *people* to distinguish them from other people. Third, in the examples of nonrestrictive clauses, it is already known which *book* and which *Moores* are being written about when the clause appears. Note that nonrestrictive clauses can be cut without sacrificing the clarity of sentences and that restrictive clauses cannot.

PUNCTUATE NONRESTRICTIVE CLAUSES

Restrictive clauses never are set off by punctuation; nonrestrictive clauses always are.

INCORRECT		CORRECT
The main problem which remarkably few writers are aware of is that of failing to set off a nonrestrictive clause by punctuation—whether by commas, dashes, or parentheses.	CHANGE TO	The main problem, which remarkably few writers are aware of, is that of failing to set off a nonrestrictive clause by punctuation—whether by commas, dashes, or parentheses.

Writers who remember the first comma sometimes forget to put in the second.

WATCH CLAUSES THAT DO NOT FOLLOW THE NOUN THEY MODIFY

Take this fragment as the problem: "The meaning of the sentence, which usually is obvious from. . . ." How can you make it clear that the relative clause relates not to *sentence,* which it follows, but to *meaning?* Here are some solutions.

Make the object of the prepositional phrase plural and rely on verb number

The meaning of the sentence, which usually is obvious from . . .	TRY	The meaning of sentences, which usually is obvious from . . .

Repeat the noun before a relative clause

The meaning of the sentence, which usually is obvious from . . .	TRY	The meaning of the sentence, meaning which usually is obvious from . . .

Delete the intervening prepositional phrase

The meaning of the sentence, which usually is obvious from . . .	TRY	The meaning, which usually is obvious from . . .

Rewrite the sentence

The meaning of the sentence, which usually is obvious from . . .	TRY	The meaning of sentences usually is obvious from . . .

AVOID HOPSCOTCHING BETWEEN THAT AND WHICH

Many writers think a sentence is made more elegant by a restrictive clause introduced by *which*. But the usage that Fowler, Follett, Strunk and White, and many other arbiters of usage prefer is to use *that* for restrictive clauses, *which* for nonrestrictive. Such usage at least shows that the writer knows the difference between restrictive and nonrestrictive clauses.

ACCEPTABLE		PREFERRED
The book which I wrote in 1981 is about French politics.	CHANGE TO	The book that I wrote in 1981 is about French politics.

The use of *that* leaves no question about whether the clause is restrictive. And by reserving *which* for nonrestrictive clauses, there is no question about which *which* clauses are to be punctuated. Note, however, the exception of restrictive clauses that begin with a preposition: *the manner in which she does things.* Note, too, that the exception can be circumvented by rewriting: *the way she does things.*

AVOID TOO MANY THAT'S, WHICH'S, AND WHO'S

A sentence or paragraph can have too many *that*'s, as adjectives, conjunctions, relative pronouns, demonstrative pronouns, and other parts of speech. A sentence can also have too many *which*'s and *who*'s. Here are some common solutions.

Cut out "that is" and "that are" (and "who is" and "who are")

Cars that are sold after January will not have a six-month warranty.	CHANGE TO	Cars sold after January will not have a six-month warranty.

People who are living in   CHANGE TO   People living in glass
glass houses should   houses should draw the
draw the blinds.   blinds.

Cut out "which is" and "which are" (and "who is" and "who are")

A good solution, which   CHANGE TO   A good solution, known
is known as ellipsis, is to   as ellipsis, is to delete
delete the *which* and the   the *which* and the auxil-
auxiliary verb—which is   iary verb—a solution
a solution that works   that works best with *is*
best with *is* and *are*.   and *are*.

The king, who is   CHANGE TO   The king, twenty-one
twenty-one today, will   today, will give up his
give up his throne.   throne.

Cut out unimportant nonrestrictive clauses

Decide whether a nonre-   TRY   Decide whether a nonrestrictive clause can be cut,   strictive clause can be cut.
which often is the fate it
deserves.

Raise the nonrestrictive clause to a main or subordinate clause

Most nonrestrictive clauses are unimportant, but if they are not, raise
them to a main or subordinate clause.

Nonrestrictive clauses,   TRY   Nonrestrictive clauses
which sometimes carry ideas   sometimes carry ideas
important to the flow of   important to the flow of
argument, should some-   argument and should sometimes be raised to the status   times be raised to the status
of a main clause.   of a main clause.

Nonrestrictive clauses,   TRY   If nonrestrictive clauses
which sometimes carry ideas   carry ideas important to the
important to the flow of   flow of argument, they
argument, should some-   should sometimes be raised
times be raised to the status   to the status of a subordi-
of a main clause.   nate clause.

Chapter *8* The Active Voice

If the subject acts, the voice is active. If the subject is acted on, the voice is passive. The red flag for the passive voice is some variation of an auxiliary verb *(was, will be, have been, is being),* plus a past participle *(built, written, directed),* plus *by* if the actor is mentioned.

PASSIVE VOICE	ACTIVE VOICE
This book was written by me.	I wrote this book.
I was given an advance by the publisher.	The publisher gave me an advance.
It was planned that the book would be published (by them) in the fall of 1982.	W. W. Norton planned to publish the book in the fall of 1982.

Voice thus gives a choice. Too few writers take it, however, relying instead on the flaccid passive, which almost always takes more words. The active voice normally is shorter, livelier, and more direct—and so is usually preferred.

SWITCHING FROM PASSIVE VOICE TO ACTIVE

There are two usual ways of switching from the passive voice to the active. One is to transpose the subject and the object, cutting out the passive baggage in the bargain. The other is to give the sentence an active subject.

PASSIVE VOICE		ACTIVE VOICE

Transpose the subject and the object

| The bill will have to be approved by Congress. | CHANGE TO | Congress will have to approve the bill. |
| That book was written by Tom Wolfe. | CHANGE TO | Tom Wolfe wrote that book. |

Give the sentence an active subject

The book was written in 1981.	CHANGE TO	She wrote the book in 1981.
The tire will have to be changed.	CHANGE TO	You will have to change the tire.
It is expected . . .	TRY	We expect . . .
It is felt . . .	TRY	I feel . . .
It is thought . . .	TRY	Many people think . . .
It will be remembered that . . .	TRY	Remember that . . .

In making the impersonal personal, avoid the use of *one*, which is equally impersonal. If used more than once, it sounds overworked: *One wants to avoid having one's sentences sound overworked, doesn't one?*

WHEN TO USE THE PASSIVE VOICE

Some rule-mongers would say that the passive voice should never be used (or, would say that you should never use the passive voice). True, it generally is better to use the active voice because it is more direct and more concise. But the subject of the sentence should dictate voice. At issue is whether the subject of the sentence is the subject of the paragraph.

The passive has two justifiable uses, both of which turn on whether the actor is less important than what is acted on.

If the actor should be left out

| I manipulated the variables to see if the direction of causation could be determined. | CHANGE TO | The variables were manipulated to determine the direction of causation. |

The Department of Commerce of the United States government increased the incentives to encourage producers to export.

CHANGE TO

Incentives were increased to encourage producers to export.

If what is acted on is the subject of the rest of the paragraph

Stockman, because of his experience in Congress, knows the budget. But the President will probably ask him to resign.

CHANGE TO

Stockman, because of his experience in Congress, knows the budget. But he will probably be asked to resign.

Chapter 9 **Parallel Constructions**

Words and groups of words that do the same work are easier to read if they are similar (parallel) in grammatical construction.

NOT PARALLEL		PARALLEL
Aides on Capitol Hill talk about running the country and the manipulation of constituents.	CHANGE TO	Aides on Capitol Hill talk about running the country and manipulating constituents.
Anita is responsible for editing and handling many aspects of production.	CHANGE TO	Anita is responsible for editing and for handling many aspects of production.

One red flag for the sameness of function is a coordinating conjunction—an *and, but, for,* or *nor*—which by definition joins words, phrases, and clauses that have the same function or similar functions. Another red flag is a pair of correlative conjunctions: *both—and; either—or; whether—or; not only—but also.* The words and groups of words that follow each of the pair should also be parallel in construction. The construction of sentences presenting similar facts or ideas should be parallel, too, as should any recurring sentence parts.

PARALLELISM WITH COORDINATING CONJUNCTIONS

the mama bear, the papa bear, and their young cub.	CHANGE TO	the mama bear, the papa bear, and the baby bear.
Do not fold, put on a spindle, or mutilate.	CHANGE TO	Do not fold, spindle, or mutilate.
He entered gingerly, she with recklessness.	CHANGE TO	He entered gingerly, she recklessly.
savings accounts, treasury bills, and the money-market certificate.	CHANGE TO	savings accounts, treasury bills, and money-market certificates.
new ways of planting seed and to grow corn.	CHANGE TO	new ways of planting seed and growing corn.
the plumber's wrench, carpenter's hammer, and the pen of the writer.	CHANGE TO	the plumber's wrench, the carpenter's hammer, and the writer's pen.
the good, the bad, and ugly.	CHANGE TO	the good, the bad, and the ugly.
the excesses of the 1960s, selfishness of the 1970s, and the bitterness that characterizes this decade.	CHANGE TO	the excesses of the 60s, the selfishness of the 70s, and the bitterness of the 80s.
developed countries and the developing countries.	CHANGE TO	developed countries and developing countries.
	OR	the developed countries and the developing countries.
schoolchildren and the parent.	CHANGE TO	schoolchildren and parents.
	OR	the schoolchild and the parent.

PARALLELISM WITH CORRELATIVE CONJUNCTIONS

Neither a borrower, nor a person who borrows money be.	CHANGE TO	Neither a borrower, nor a lender be.

The sale of the AWACs   CHANGE TO   The sale of the AWACs
was opposed both by   was opposed both by
Israel and the Jewish   Israel and by the Jewish
lobby in the United   lobby in the United
States.   States.

Elements often are not parallel because one of the correlatives is out
of place.

Solving the problem   CHANGE TO   Solving the problem
requires that you both   requires both that you
recognize it and that you   recognize it and that you
do something about it.   do something about it.

Chapter 10 **Consistency**

Consistency is one of the main things an editor looks for in a piece of writing, consistency in the style of spelling, of punctuation, and of writing numbers as words or figures. To be inconsistent is to be sloppy—say, by alternating between travelled and traveled, 10 and ten, or % and percent. So, above all, be consistent, even if eccentric. The idea is to pick one style and to stick to it. The best way to keep track of the styles you have chosen is to write them on a style sheet (see chapter 11).

In the examples that follow, the styles consistently chosen in the right-hand column reflect the preferences of most editors today. In most of the examples, it would have been acceptable (but not preferable) to have consistently chosen the alternative style.

SPELLING

Follow the style of spelling and the first entries of different acceptable spellings in the eighth edition of *Webster's New Collegiate Dictionary,* the dictionary most editors use.

INCONSISTENT   CONSISTENT

Words with two or more acceptable spellings

sizable on one page, and *sizeable* on the next	CHANGE TO	*sizable* on one page, and *sizable* on the next

traveling on one page, and *travelling* on the next	CHANGE TO	*traveling* on one page, and *traveling* on the next

Different words serving one function

nonetheless on one page, and *nevertheless, none the less,* or *never the less* on the next	CHANGE TO	*nonetheless* on one page, and *nonetheless* on the next
Second, on one page, and *Secondly,* on the next	CHANGE TO	*Second,* on one page, and *Second,* on the next

Latin plurals

formulas on one page, and *formulae* on the next	CHANGE TO	*formulas* on one page, and *formulas* on the next

OPEN, SOLID, AND HYPHENATED TERMS

Consult a dictionary to find out the accepted spelling of compound nouns, whether open *(field worker)*, solid *(fieldworker)*, or hyphenated *(field-worker)*. Hyphenate compound adjectives *(long-term gains),* unless they are recognizable as paired adjectives that usually modify the noun they are in front of *(current account deficit)*. Run prefixes solid (without a hyphen), unless such curiosities as *crosssectional* are the result, or unless the prefix is attached to a compound word *(non-oil-exporting)* or a capitalized word *(non-British)*.

INCONSISTENT		CONSISTENT

Prefixes

antismoking on one page, and *anti-smoking* on the next	CHANGE TO	*antismoking* on one page, and *antismoking* on the next
nonviolent on one page, and *non-violent* on the next	CHANGE TO	*nonviolent* on one page, and *nonviolent* on the next

Compound nouns

cost-effectiveness on one page, and *cost effectiveness* on the next	CHANGE TO	*cost-effectiveness* on one page, and *cost-effectiveness* on the next
decision-making on one page, and *decision making* on the next	CHANGE TO	*decision-making* on one page, and *decision-making* on the next

Compound adjectives

low-income groups on one page, and *low income groups* on the next	CHANGE TO	*low-income groups* on one page, and *low-income groups* on the next
short-term gains on one page, and *short term gains* on the next	CHANGE TO	*short-term gains* on one page, and *short-term gains* on the next

CAPITALS

If you have a choice of using a capital or a small letter, use the small letter. Use capitals only when you must, never for emphasis.

INCONSISTENT		CONSISTENT
in figure 2 on one page, and *in Figure 2* on the next	CHANGE TO	*in figure 2* on one page, and *in figure 2* on the next
the president on one page, and *the President* on the next	CHANGE TO	*the president* on one page, and *the president* on the next
the project on one page, and *the Project* on the next	CHANGE TO	*the project* on one page, and *the project* on the next

SYMBOLS AND ABBREVIATIONS

The preferred practice is to avoid symbols and abbreviations. An exception is to use symbols for currencies in numerals *($400)*.

INCONSISTENT		CONSISTENT
Symbols		
percent on one page, and % on the next	CHANGE TO	*percent* on one page, and *percent* on the next
ten degrees on one page, and *10°* on the next	CHANGE TO	*ten degrees* on one page, and *ten degrees* on the next
Abbreviations of units		
kilometers on one page, and *km.* on the next	CHANGE TO	*kilometers* on one page, and *kilometers* on the next

square feet on one page, and *sq. ft.* on the next	CHANGE TO	*square feet* on one page, and *square feet* on the next

Abbreviations of Latin terms

and so on on one page, and *etc.* on the next	CHANGE TO	*and so on* on one page, and *and so on* on the next
that is, on one page, and *i.e.,* on the next	CHANGE TO	*that is,* on one page, and *that is,* on the next

Other abbreviations

months on one page, and *mos.* on the next	CHANGE TO	*months* on one page, and *months* on the next

INITIALS

The main problem with initials is that they are overused. If you must use them, spell the words they represent on their first appearance, followed by the initials in parentheses [*the gross national product (GNP)*], and then use initials. Initials read one-by-one are preceded by an article *(the GNP);* those read as a word are not *(OPEC)*.

INCONSISTENT		CONSISTENT
by OPEC on one page, and *by the OPEC* on the next	CHANGE TO	*by OPEC* on one page, and *by OPEC* on the next
of the GNP on one page, and *of GNP* on the next	CHANGE TO	*of the GNP* on one page, and *of the GNP* on the next
the United States on one page, and *the U.S.* on the next	CHANGE TO	*the United States* on one page, and *the United States* on the next

NUMBERS

One style is to use words for single-digit numbers and to use numerals for all others; another is to use words for single-digit and double-digit numbers and to use numerals for all others. Percentages should nonetheless be written as numerals *(2 percent);* large rough numbers as words *(a million);* large precise numbers as a combination of numerals and words *(1.3 billion)*. There naturally are other views.

Some editors recommend the use of figures all the time; others, the use of words, even for three million four hundred ninety thousand dollars. Whatever the system you adopt, be consistent.

INCONSISTENT		CONSISTENT
two cars on one page, and *2 cars* on the next	CHANGE TO	*two cars* on one page, and *two cars* on the next
the first on one page, and *the 1st* on the next	CHANGE TO	*the first* on one page, and *the first* on the next
eleven o'clock on one page, and *11 o'clock* on the next	CHANGE TO	*eleven o'clock* on one page, and *eleven o'clock* on the next
1950s on one page, and *50's, 1950's, fifties, Fifties, nineteen fifties, or Nineteen Fifties* on the next	CHANGE TO	*1950s* on one page, and *1950s* on the next
1981–82 on one page, and *1981–1982* on the next	CHANGE TO	*1981–82* on one page, and *1981–82* on the next
0.5 on one page, and *.5* on the next	CHANGE TO	*0.5* on one page, and *0.5* on the next
two-thirds on one page, and *⅔* on the next	CHANGE TO	*two-thirds* on one page, and *two-thirds* on the next

PUNCTUATION

The main incidents of inconsistency in punctuation are with series, with introductory phrases, and with quotation marks.

INCONSISTENT		CONSISTENT
the apples, oranges, and pears on one page, and *the apples, oranges and pears* on the next	CHANGE TO	*the apples, oranges, and pears* on one page, and *the apples, oranges, and pears* on the next
France, Germany, and Switzerland on one page, and *France, Germany and Switzerland* on the next	CHANGE TO	*France, Germany, and Switzerland* on one page, and *France, Germany, and Switzerland* on the next

In 1970 the Russians . . . on one page, and *In 1970, the Russians . . .* on the next	CHANGE TO	*In 1970 the Russians . . .* on one page, and *In 1970 the Russians . . .* on the next
After the war they . . . on one page, and *After the war, they . . .* on the next	CHANGE TO	*After the war they . . .* on one page, and *After the war they . . .* on the next
the "health gap." on one page, and *the "health gap".* on the next	CHANGE TO	*the "health gap."* on one page, and *the "health gap."* on the next

Chapter *11* **Basic Tools**

Two important things in writing are to continue learning and to find answers to questions. The two go hand in hand, and to help you do them you need some basic tools.

Dictionary

Keep a dictionary within reach when you are writing or editing. Many editors use the eighth edition of *Webster's New Collegiate Dictionary* (Springfield, Mass.: G. & C. Merriam Company, 1977).

- Use it to find out what words mean and to confirm that words mean what you think they mean.
- Use it to find out the preferred spelling of a word.
- Use it to see a word in context: *dialectical,* a ~ philosopher.
- Use it to find out what preposition to use: *methodical,* ~ in his daily routine.
- Use it to see how seeming synonyms can be differentiated. For example, see the entry for *masterful* in *Webster's Dictionary* to see how that word can be differentiated from *domineering, imperious,* and *peremptory.*

A dictionary also helps in finding the accepted spelling of the names of people and places. And many dictionaries have a section on style and punctuation (*Webster's Dictionary*, pp. 1515–27).

Style sheet

To be consistent in spelling, punctuation, hyphenation, capitalization, and writing numbers in words or numerals, keep a style sheet. Indispensable for writing by one person, and imperative for writing by more than one person, a style sheet is a simple tool that can save time and avoid confusion (see the sample on page 43). It is made by drawing a few lines on a sheet of typing paper and writing groups of initials in each box. Each time you write or see a word that has more than one acceptable style, write it in the appropriate box; for example, write *decision-making* in the ABCD box, *traveling* in the QRST box. Then when you run into these words elsewhere, you can check the style against the style sheet (rather than having to flip through all the pages to see how you spelled them the first time). For long pieces it often helps to keep a style sheet for each of the main areas of inconsistency: one for spelling (especially that of names and terms), one for hyphens, one for capitals, one for numbers, and one for initials.

Checklist

You should check the use and usefulness of each word, phrase, sentence, paragraph, and section. If you do not have the time for such a task, at least check a few basic things.

- Check all spelling, hyphens, capitals, numbers, and important names and terms against your style sheet.
- Make a table of contents to identify problems of organization and to help your readers.
- Underline and try to rectify long sentences, awkward sentences, passive verbs, and constructions that should be parallel but are not.
- Check that subjects and verbs agree in number.
- Check that all *who* and *which* clauses are correctly punctuated.
- Check that all introductory clauses beginning with an *-ing* word relate to what immediately follows.
- Check that pairs, series, and compound subjects and predicates are arranged from short to long, from simple to compound.
- Cut what is of little use.
- Proofread everything you send out. A list of proofreader's marks is under *proofreader* in *Webster's Dictionary*.

SAMPLE STYLE SHEET

ABCD	EFGH
antismoking	(the) executive director
busing	formulas (pl.)
benefited	figure 1
channeling	
cooperate	
cost-effectiveness	
decision-making	

IJKL	MNOP
	midproject
	multidisciplinary
	nonviolent
	percent
	(the) project

QRST	UVWXYZ
sizable	
short-term (adj.)	
table 1	
traveling	
tradable	

NUMBERS

1980s	2 million
mid-1970s	1,215
1980–81	first
$400	eleven o'clock
two cars	three-quarters
2 percent	
two percentage points	

INITIALS, NAMES, AND IMPORTANT TERMS

BOAL=	basic organization of associated labor
IPO project=	Improved Pregnancy Outcome Project
GDP=	gross domestic product

Part II **WHAT EDITORS CUT,
CHANGE, AND COMPARE**

The recommendations in this part are just that: recommendations. But nine times out of ten, the recommendations will give you a sentence that is more clear, more concise, and obviously the product of a careful writer. The recommendations do not always work, but if they do not, they may point to other problems that call for another try at writing the sentence. The idea underlying the brevity and precision proposed here is to throw attention on the words and phrases that deserve attention in a sentence.

The recommendations CUT and CHANGE TO indicate cuts and changes that almost always are preferred because they trim fat or because they avoid words and phrases that are overused, are long when they could be short, or depart from current usage. The recommendations TRY and TRY TO CUT indicate changes and cuts that you should consider because they are preferred in many instances, but not all. The recommendation COMPARE indicates a choice to be made depending on the meaning and context. In phrases that are alphabetically placed according to words other than the first, the preceding word or words are enclosed by parentheses: for example, *(for the) purpose of* is placed under *p*.

The brackets after an entry enclose information either to help define a word or to identify what part of speech a word is: for example, *adverse* [*bad, unfavorable*] and *accord* [*the verb*]. Recommendations for the treatment of Latin words, phrases, and abbreviations are drawn together at the end.

A	**A**	**A**
a	COMPARE	an

Before *h*, *a* is preferred if the *h* is voiced, as in *a hotel*, and
an if it is not, as in *an hour*.

a, an [general]	COMPARE	the [particular]

The article *a (an)* goes before an indefinite one of a class, as
in *a book;* the article *the* before a definite one of a class, as in
the book.
No article is used for all of a class, as in *books;* but *the* is
used for some of a class, as in *the books of X.*
A tendency, not to be indulged, is to drop *the* before singular constructions that are followed by a prepositional
phrase:
practice of family planning should be *the practice of family
planning.*

a lot of	CHANGE TO	much, many
(in) abeyance	CHANGE TO	held up
absolutely	CUT	
accomplish	TRY	do
accord [the verb]	TRY	give
(in) accordance with	TRY	by, under, in accord with
accordingly	TRY TO CUT OR TRY	so, therefore
(take into) account	COMPARE	take account of
(on) account of	CHANGE TO	caused by, because of
achieve	TRY	do, get, reach
acquaint	TRY	tell, inform
acquiesce with	CHANGE TO	acquiesce to
acquire	TRY	get
action	TRY	act
(take) action	CHANGE TO	act
active(ly)	CUT	
actual(ly)	CUT	
(in) addition	TRY	and, also
(in) addition to	CHANGE TO	besides
additional	CHANGE TO	more
additionally	CHANGE TO	and, also

adjacent to	CHANGE TO	near, next to, close to
administrate	CHANGE TO	administer
admit of [leave possibility for]	COMPARE	admit
admit to (something)	CHANGE TO	admit (something)
admittance [permission for access to a physical space]	COMPARE	admission [all other uses]
adventuresome	CHANGE TO	adventurous
adverse [bad, unfavorable]	COMPARE	averse [opposed, disinclined]
advert to	CHANGE TO	refer to
advise	TRY	tell, inform
advocate that	CHANGE TO	advocate
affect [the verb: influence]	COMPARE	effect [the verb: bring about], effect [the noun: result]
affirmative	TRY	yes
afford [the verb]	CHANGE TO	give
(the) aforementioned ~	CHANGE TO	that ~, those ~s
against	TRY	compared with
aggravate	CHANGE TO	annoy, make worse
agree on, to, and with	CHANGE TO	agree on a course of action, agree to terms proposed, agree with an adversary
albeit	CHANGE TO	though, although
all [the adjective]	TRY TO CUT	
all of	CHANGE TO	all
all together [collectively]	COMPARE	altogether [completely]
allows for	CHANGE TO	allows
allude [refer indirectly]	COMPARE	refer [directly]
allusion [indirect reference]	COMPARE	reference [direct]
allusion [indirect reference]	COMPARE	delusion [deception of belief], illusion [visual deception or false perception]
alongside of	CHANGE TO	alongside

already has been	TRY	has been
alright [not a word]	CHANGE TO	all right
Also, . . .	CHANGE TO	And . . . , . . .
		also . . .

Most editors would change *Also, I fell ill* to *And I fell ill* or *I
also fell ill.*

(and) also	CHANGE TO	and
alter(ation)	CHANGE TO	change
alternate(ly) [by turns]	COMPARE	alternative(ly) [of choice]
alternative [the adjective]	CHANGE TO	other, different

Let *alternative* stand as an adjective if it refers to a choice
between two or more things.

alternative [the noun]	TRY	choice
alternative(ly) [of choice]	COMPARE	alternate(ly) [by turns]
although	TRY	but, though
altogether [completely]	COMPARE	all together [collectively]
ameliorate	CHANGE TO	improve
amidst	CHANGE TO	amid
among [three or more]	COMPARE	between [two or two at a time]

The conventional practice is to reserve *between* for two,
among for three or more.
Thus: *The winnings were divided between the two of them* or
among the three of them.
But *between* is used for three or more if what is described
applies to two at a time. Thus: *Trade between western
nations.*

amongst	CHANGE TO	among
(the) amount of ~	CHANGE TO	the ~
an historical	CHANGE TO	a historical
analogous	CHANGE TO	similar
and also	TRY	and
~ and/or ~	CHANGE TO	~ and ~ ~ or ~

anterior to	CHANGE TO	before
anticipate that	CHANGE TO	expect that
antipathy for	CHANGE TO	antipathy to or toward
any	TRY TO CUT	
apart from	TRY	except for
(it is) apparent that	CUT	
(it) appears that	CUT	
appears to be	COMPARE	is
append	CHANGE TO	add
apprise	CHANGE TO	tell, inform
approach [the noun]	TRY	way, method
approbation [praise for an act]	COMPARE	approval [praise for general behavior]
appropriate	TRY	right, proper
approval [praise for general behavior]	COMPARE	approbation [praise for an act]
approximately	COMPARE	about, roughly

If something has been mathematically approximated, use
approximately.
If a precise figure is being rounded or if an imprecise figure
is being glossed, use *about* or *roughly*.

are	COMPARE	is

Such pronouns as *each, none, either,* and *neither* are singular
and call for a singular verb: *each of them is; none of them is;
either of the two is; neither of the two is.*
Some writers and editors use a plural verb if the sense of
the pronoun is collective, or if there is an intervening prepositional phrase with a plural object, as in *neither of them are
coming.*
It is recommended here that you use the singular verb
unless you have a good reason for using the plural.
Whatever the choice, be consistent.

are ~ing	TRY

The construction of *are* plus a present participle is often
used unnecessarily: *The farmers are producing corn and beans*
is often written when the meaning is *The farmers produce
corn and beans.*

(in the) area of ~	TRY	in ~
arising from the fact that	CHANGE TO	because
arguable	CHANGE TO	can be argued that, can be questioned whether
around 20 percent	CHANGE TO	about 20 percent
As	CHANGE TO	If, When, Since, Because
as	COMPARE	like

The use of *as* and *like* is muddied by misuse in speech, misuse that should not invade writing.
A simple distinction covering most cases is to reserve *as* for
constructions that have a verb, *like* for those that do not.
Thus: *She acts like a child; she acts as a child would act.*
This distinction does not apply to constructions with a verb
in a modifying clause: *The children in the community, like
children that live anywhere in the Third World, . . .*

(such) as	COMPARE	like

In introducing examples, use *such as* rather than *like:*
*Some countries, such as Poland (not: like Poland), are overex-
tended in their external debt.*
Reserve *like* for likenesses:
Brazil, like Poland, may be overextended in its external debt.

as a result of	CHANGE TO	from, because of
as follow	CHANGE TO	as follows
as if	COMPARE	like

Reserve *as if* for constructions that can stand as sentences,
like for those that cannot.
Thus: *It looks as if I may be fired; it looks like another month of
heavy layoffs.*

as long as	COMPARE	so long as

Purists reserve *as long as* for positive constructions, *so long
as* for negative:
As long as you succeed but *So long as you do not fail.*

as of	CHANGE TO	starting, beginning
as per	CHANGE TO	on, for, about, further to, in accord with
as regards	CHANGE TO	on, for, about
(~) as such	CHANGE TO	~
as to	TRY TO CUT OR CHANGE TO	in, of, on, for, about
as to whether (or why, how, what, who)	CHANGE TO	whether (or why, how, what, who)
as well as	TRY	and, also
assist(ance)	TRY	help
assure [someone that]	COMPARE	ensure [that], insure [something]
assuredly	CUT	
at constant (or current) prices	CHANGE TO	in constant (or current) prices
at the end of	TRY	after
attain	TRY	get or gain
attempt	TRY	try
autarchy [sovereignty]	COMPARE	autarky [self-sufficiency]
author [as a verb]	CHANGE TO	write
available [a word to avoid]	TRY TO CUT	
averse [opposed, disinclined]	COMPARE	adverse [bad, unfavorable]

B	**B**	**B**
(date, refer, or return) back	TRY	date (or refer or return)
(the) balance	TRY	the rest, remainder
based on	CHANGE TO	by, for, from, because of
Based on ~, . . .	TRY	~ shows that
(on an annual) basis	CHANGE TO	yearly, annually, once a year
(on a regular) basis	CHANGE TO	regularly
(on a year-to-year) basis	CHANGE TC	year to year

(on the) basis of	CHANGE TO	by, on, for, from, because of
be [the subjunctive verb]	TRY	is, are, should be
be helpful	CHANGE TO	help
(is) because	CHANGE TO	is that, is caused by, is attributable to
(the reason is) because	CHANGE TO	the reason is that
begin	TRY	start
(the issue) being addressed is	CHANGE TO	the issue is
believe [for convictions]	COMPARE	feel [for emotions], think [for speculations]
benefits	TRY	benefit
beside [next to]	COMPARE	besides [except, in addition]
bestow	TRY	give
between [two or two at a time]	COMPARE	among [three or more]

See the comments under *among*.

between 1970–80	CHANGE TO	during 1970–80, between 1970 and 1980
biannually	CHANGE TO	every two years, twice a year
bimonthly	CHANGE TO	every two months, twice a month
biweekly	CHANGE TO	every two weeks, twice a week
bored with	CHANGE TO	bored by
both	TRY TO CUT OR TRY	they, the two
both of them are	CHANGE TO	they are
but	COMPARE	and

It often happens that *but* is used when *and* would be better
or even correct, especially in joining independent clauses
that are not contradictory or exceptional.
A good practice is to try replacing *but* by *and*.

but rather	CHANGE TO	but
but + however	CHANGE TO	But, however
by itself	CHANGE TO	alone
by means of	CHANGE TO	by

(rose or fell) by 2 per-cent	CHANGE TO	rose (or fell) 2 percent
by virtue of	CHANGE TO	by
by way of ~ing	CHANGE TO	to ~

C   C   C

can [ability]	COMPARE	may [permission], might [possibility]
cannot help but	CHANGE TO	can only
capability	TRY	ability
capacity	COMPARE	ability, capability

Reserve *capacity* for volumes and amounts, *ability* and *capability* for what can be done.
Thus: *The capacity of the container is ten gallons.*
The capacity of the machine is 1,000 units a day.
The machine has the ability to produce several products.
People have *abilities,* not *capacities.*

capital [of column or country]	COMPARE	Capitol [building]
careful(ly)	TRY TO CUT	
case [a word to avoid]	TRY TO CUT	

Misused, overused, and otherwise abused, the word *case* has at least six acceptable uses: *a case of yellow fever, you have no case, in case of need, a case of burglary, a law case, the case of Quiller-Couch against case.* The examples here are borrowed from Gowers, who borrowed them from Fowler.
A seventh acceptable use is the main use: *a case of beer.*
But note in the following lines how many constructions that use *case* can be shortened.

(in that) case	TRY	then
(in the) case of	TRY TO CUT OR TRY	by, in, of, for
(than is the) case with ~	CHANGE TO	than with ~
(in) cases in which	CHANGE TO	if, when
category	TRY	class, group
cater for	CHANGE TO	cater to
cease	TRY	stop
ceiling	TRY	limit, maximum

center around	TRY	center on
(a) certain ~	TRY	a ~
certainly	CUT	
(is of a ~) character	CHANGE TO	is ~

For example: *The house is of a rustic character* should be *The house is rustic.*

(~ in) character	CHANGE TO	~

For example: *The food is mild in character* should be *The food is mild.*

(~ of this) character	CHANGE TO	~ such as, ~ like this
clearly	CUT	
coauthor [the verb]	CHANGE TO	write with
cognizant	CHANGE TO	aware
combines ~ with ~	TRY	combines ~ and ~
commence	CHANGE TO	start, begin
commencement	CHANGE TO	start, beginning
common [of many]	COMPARE	mutual [reciprocated]
comparable to	TRY	the same as
comparatively	TRY TO CUT	
compare to [liken]	COMPARE	compare with [set side by side]
(in) comparison to	CHANGE TO	in comparison with
compensate (compensation)	TRY	pay, reward
complete	TRY	finish
component	CHANGE TO	part
compose [constitute, make up]	COMPARE	consist of [comprise, is made up of]

Accepted usage is this: *The team is made up of (or consists of or comprises) nine players; nine players make up (or compose or constitute) the team.*

Constitute and *comprise* should be reserved for scholarly writing.

comprise [consist of, is made up of]	COMPARE	constitute	[compose, make up]

See the comments under *compose.*

comprise [all parts]	COMPARE	include [some parts]
conceal	TRY	hide
(the) concept of ~	CHANGE TO	~
(so far as ~ is) concerned	CHANGE TO	for ~
(where ~ is) concerned	CHANGE TO	for ~
(the ~) concerned are	CHANGE TO	the ~ are
concerning	CHANGE TO	at, of, on, for, about
(the) conclusions reached	CHANGE TO	the conclusions
confident of	CHANGE TO	sure of, sure that
conform with	CHANGE TO	conform to
(in this) connection	CHANGE TO	about
(in) connection with	CHANGE TO	on, for, about
connote [signify attributes of a word]	COMPARE	denote [define meaning of a word]

The word *table* usually *denotes* a raised surface on legs; it can *connote* dining.

(general) consensus	CHANGE TO	consensus
consensus of opinion	CHANGE TO	consensus
consequently	TRY	so, therefore
consider	TRY	think about
considerable	TRY TO CUT	
(take into) consideration	CHANGE TO	consider
consist of [is made up of]	COMPARE	compose [make up]

See the comments under *compose*.

constant 1975 prices	CHANGE TO	1975 prices
(at) constant prices	CHANGE TO	in constant prices
constitute [compose, make up]	COMPARE	comprise [consist of, is made up of]

See the comments under *compose*.

constructive(ly)	TRY TO CUT	
contained	TRY	had
contained in	TRY	in
contemptible [deserving scorn]	COMPARE	contemptuous [scornful]

contemptuous [scornful]	COMPARE	contemptible [deserving scorn]
contend for, with, against	CHANGE TO	contend for ideals, contend with neighbors, contend against bad weather
contiguous with	CHANGE TO	contiguous to
continual [recurring with interruptions]	COMPARE	continuous [occurring without interruption]

The flow of water is continuous; the dripping of water is continual.

continuous [occurring without interruption]	COMPARE	continual [recurring with interruptions]
(on the) contrary	TRY	no
(to the) contrary	TRY	not so
(a) contrast of X and Y	CHANGE TO	a contrast between X and Y
contrast to [the verb]	CHANGE TO	contrast with
(in) contrast with	CHANGE TO	in contrast to
(a) contrast with Y	CHANGE TO	a contrast to Y
contribute to	TRY	add to
converse	COMPARE	obverse, reverse

Consider the statement: *All authors are good writers.*
The *converse* is:
Some good writers are authors.
The *obverse* is:
No authors are bad authors.
The *converse* and *obverse* are each the *reverse* of the first statement.

convince [someone of, that]	COMPARE	persuade [someone of, to, that]

There is much overlap except before *to*, where only *persuade* will do.
You can *persuade* or *convince* someone *of* the wisdom of a policy;
you can *persuade* or *convince* someone *that* a policy is wise;

you can *persuade* (but not *convince*) someone *to* adopt
a policy.

cooperate together with	CHANGE TO	cooperate with
(with the) cooperation of	TRY	with the help of
correspond with [by letter]	COMPARE	correspond to [match, go with]
costs [the noun]	TRY	cost
(of) course	CUT	
credence [trust, belief]	COMPARE	credibility [of being believable], credulity [of readiness to believe]
credible [believable]	COMPARE	creditable [deserving credit], credulous [willing to believe]
critical	TRY TO CUT	
crucial	TRY TO CUT	
culminate with	CHANGE TO	culminate in
cultivatable	CHANGE TO	cultivable
cum	CHANGE TO	and, with
(at) current prices	CHANGE TO	in current prices
currently	CUT OR CHANGE TO	now

D	**D**	**D**
data is	CHANGE TO	data are
date back to	CHANGE TO	date to
decide about this	CHANGE TO	decide this
decidedly	CUT	
(make a) decision	CHANGE TO	decide
decisions made by	CHANGE TO	decisions by
decrease [the noun or intransitive verb]	CHANGE TO	drop, fall
decrease [the transitive verb]	TRY	cut, reduce, shorten
defective [of quality]	COMPARE	deficient [of quantity]
deficient [of quantity]	COMPARE	defective [of quality]
definite(ly)	TRY TO CUT	
definitive [final, conclusive]	COMPARE	definite [decided, explicit]
(the) degree of ~	CHANGE TO	the ~

delusion [deception of belief]	COMPARE	allusion [indirect reference], illusion [visual deception or false perception]
demonstrate	TRY	show
denote [define meaning of a word]	COMPARE	connote [signify attributes of a word]

See the comments under *connote*.

depend(ing) upon	CHANGE TO	depend(ing) on
(examine in) depth	CHANGE TO	examine
desiderata	CHANGE TO	desired things
desire	TRY	want, wish
(is) desirous of	CHANGE TO	wants
desist	CHANGE TO	stop
despite the fact that	CHANGE TO	although
determine	TRY	test, study, decide, find out
devoid of	CHANGE TO	without
did [as intensifier]	TRY TO CUT	

For example: *did provide* usually should be *provided*.

differ from, with, over, about	CHANGE TO	differ from something, differ with neighbors over or about the election
differ(ent) than	CHANGE TO	differ(ent) from
(in three) different ways	CHANGE TO	in three ways
differential [for math or car]	COMPARE	difference, different [for everything else]
dilemma	COMPARE	difficulty

The word *dilemma* means two horns, so it is illogical to say *horns of a dilemma*. The word should be used for a choice between two unsatisfactory things or courses of action.

dimension	TRY TO CUT	
discrepancy	TRY	difference
discreet [circumspect]	COMPARE	discrete [separate]
discrete [separate]	COMPARE	discreet [circumspect]
disassociate	CHANGE TO	dissociate

disinterested [impartial]	COMPARE	uninterested [not interested]
dispatch	TRY	send, send off
dissent with	CHANGE TO	dissent from
distinct [clear]	COMPARE	distinctive [individual]
distinctive [individual]	COMPARE	distinct [clear]
diverge(nt)	TRY	differ(ent)
divide up	CHANGE TO	divide
do [as intensifier]	TRY TO CUT	

For example: *do provide* usually should be *provide*.

donate	TRY	give
double	COMPARE	twice

Usage now seems to be to reserve *double* for the verb and *twice* for the noun, as in: *I'll double what I give you; I'll give you twice that amount.*

doubt if	TRY	doubt that
doubtless(ly)	CUT	
due to	TRY	caused by, because of
due to the fact that	CHANGE TO	because
dwell	CHANGE TO	live

E	E	E
e.g. [*exempli gratia* = by way of example]	CHANGE TO	say, for example
e.g. [for example]	COMPARE	i.e. [that is]
each and every	CHANGE TO	each, every
each of them are	CHANGE TO	each of them is
effect [the verb: bring about]	COMPARE	affect [the verb: influence], effect [the noun: result]
(have an) effect	CHANGE TO	affect
(may have the) effect of increasing	CHANGE TO	may increase
effective(ly)	TRY TO CUT	
effectuate	CHANGE TO	carry out, put into effect
(in an) effort to	CHANGE TO	to
either A, B, or C	CHANGE TO	A, B, or C
either of the three	CHANGE TO	any of the three

either of the two are	CHANGE TO	either of the two is
elapse	CHANGE TO	pass
elect [when voting]	COMPARE	choose [when choosing]
electric	COMPARE	electrical, electronic

Keep these adjectives straight by keeping in mind that *electric* and *electrical* relate to electricity, the shorter word being preferred unless it is confusing, and that *electronic* relates to electrons moving not in wires but in tubes and transistors. So: *electric clock, electrical knowledge,* and *electronic watch.*

element	TRY	part
eliminate	TRY	end, stop, cut out
elites	CHANGE TO	elite
elucidate	CHANGE TO	explain
elusive [for that sought]	COMPARE	illusory [for that gained]
emigrate to	CHANGE TO	migrate to, emigrate from
eminently	CUT	
emphasize	TRY	stress
employ	TRY	use
employment	TRY	work
encounter	TRY	meet, run into
encourage	TRY	urge
(at the) end of	TRY	after
end product	CHANGE TO	product
end result	CHANGE TO	result
endeavor [the noun and verb]	CHANGE TO	try, attempt
engage in	CHANGE TO	do, work on
enhance [heighten or increase]	TRY	make bigger, greater, or larger
enormity [outrageousness]	COMPARE	enormousness [big size, immensity]
enquire	TRY	ask
ensue	CHANGE TO	follow
ensure [that]	COMPARE	assure [someone that], insure [something]
envisage that	CHANGE TO	think that, expect that
envision	TRY	think, foresee, consider, have in mind
epigram [witty statement]	COMPARE	epigraph [quotation], epitaph [words on

		tombstone], epithet [abusive word or phrase]
equable [steady]	COMPARE	equitable [fair]
equally as	CHANGE TO	as, equally, just as
equitable [fair]	COMPARE	equable [steady]
eradicate	TRY	wipe out
ergo [= therefore]	CHANGE TO	so, thus, therefore
erstwhile	CHANGE TO	former
eschew	CHANGE TO	avoid
especially	TRY	specially
espouse	CHANGE TO	hold
essential [the adjective]	TRY TO CUT	
establish	TRY	set up, find out
et al. [*et alia* = and others]	CHANGE TO	and others
etc. [*et cetera* = and the others]	CHANGE TO	and so on, and so forth
(in the) event that	CHANGE TO	if
eventuate	CHANGE TO	occur, happen, come about
evince	CHANGE TO	show
evolve	CHANGE TO	change, develop
ex cathedra	CHANGE TO	arbitrarily
exacerbate	CHANGE TO	sharpen, make worse
examine	TRY	look at
(for) example	COMPARE	for instance

For consistency, pick one or the other and stick to it, rather than jumping back and forth between the two. The preferred usage is to reserve *example* for *for example* and *instance* for *in this instance* or *in two instances*.

(with the) exception of	CHANGE TO	except
(in) excess of	CHANGE TO	over, more than
exhibit [the verb]	TRY	show
(there) exist	CHANGE TO	there are
exists	CHANGE TO	is
(the) existence of	CUT	
existing [the adjective]	TRY TO CUT	
exit [the verb]	CHANGE TO	leave
expedite	CHANGE TO	speed up
expenditure	TRY	cost, expense, spending

expenditures	TRY	expenditure
expenses	TRY	expense
experience [the verb]	TRY	feel, have, go through
expertise	TRY	talent, know-how, knowledge
explicate	CHANGE TO	explain
expound on	CHANGE TO	expound
extant [still around]	COMPARE	extent [limit, boundary]
extend	TRY	give
extended period	TRY	long period
extent [limit, boundary]	COMPARE	extant [still around]
(the) extent of ~	CHANGE TO	the ~
(to the) extent that	CHANGE TO	as much as, so much that
extinguish	CHANGE TO	put out

F	**F**	**F**
facilitate	TRY	ease, help, make easier
facility [a word to avoid]	TRY	plant, warehouse, factory, some other specific word
(as a matter of) fact	CUT	
(the) fact remains that	CUT	
(despite the) fact that	CHANGE TO	although
(due to the) fact that	CHANGE TO	because
(in view of the) fact that	CHANGE TO	because
(the) fact that	CHANGE TO	that
factor [a word to avoid]	TRY	fact, cause, feature, element, consideration
(the ~) factor	CHANGE TO	~

For example: *The efficiency factor is important in manufacturing* should be *Efficiency is important in manufacturing.*

farther [of distance]	COMPARE	further [of time or direction]

The preference is to use *farther* when writing about physical distances: to go *farther* down the road, but to go *further* in their studies, to be *further* along in their studies, and to have a *further* step before completing their studies. Further,

of the two words, only *further* is used as a verb and as an
adverb in the sense of *moreover*.

fears [the noun]	TRY	fear
feasible [= can be done]	COMPARE	possible [= can happen]
feasible	TRY	likely, probable, plausible
feel [for emotions]	COMPARE	believe [for convictions], think [for speculations]
fell by 2 percent	CHANGE TO	fell 2 percent
female [the noun]	TRY	woman
fewer (than) [= a smaller number of]	COMPARE	less (than) [= a smaller amount of]

The preference is to use *fewer* and *fewer than* with words
that have a separate quality and can be counted, such as
persons or fence posts, and to use *less* and *less than* with
words that have a unitary quality and cannot be counted,
such as water or land.
So: *less land,* but *fewer hectares of land; less steel,* but *fewer
steel mills.*
And: *less than a quart,* but *fewer than ten quarts.*
There naturally is a middle ground filled with things that
could be considered either separate or unitary. *Years* is an
example.
So take your pick depending on whether you mean the
number of years *(fewer than ten years)* or the amount of time
(less than ten years).
And there naturally is an exception: *one less syllable.*

(in the) field of	CHANGE TO	in
figurative [metaphorical]	COMPARE	literal [exact]
filled up the ~	CHANGE TO	filled the ~
finalize	CHANGE TO	finish, complete, make final
Finally, . . .	TRY	Fourth, . . . or Fifth, . . .

Finally should be reserved for the last argument, if it is used
at all.

finance [the verb]	TRY	pay for
first began (first started or originated)	CHANGE TO	began (started or originated)
first of all	CHANGE TO	first
firstly	CHANGE TO	first
flaunt [display, show off]	COMPARE	flout [mock, scoff at]
flout [mock, scoff at]	COMPARE	flaunt [display, show off]
(as) follow	CHANGE TO	as follows
following [the preposition]	CHANGE TO	after
for example	COMPARE	for instance

See the comments under *example*.

for the purpose of	CHANGE TO	for
for the reason that	CHANGE TO	because, since
forceful [having force]	COMPARE	forcible [using force]
forcible [using force]	COMPARE	forceful [having force]
forego [go before]	COMPARE	forgo [relinquish]
(in the) foreseeable future	CHANGE TO	in the future
forgo [relinquish]	COMPARE	forego [go before]
(was in the) form of ~	CHANGE TO	was ~
(a ~ in condensed) form	CHANGE TO	a condensed ~
former [the adjective as noun]	TRY	first

Because the use of *former* and *latter* almost always forces the reader to go back to see which is which, it usually is better to repeat the antecedent. Even if the antecedent is clear, editors generally prefer to use *first* and *second*.
Never use *former* and *latter* if there are more than two antecedents: that is, do not use *former* to refer to the first of three or more antecedents, or *latter* to refer to the last of three or more.

forthwith	CHANGE TO	now, immediately
fourthly	CHANGE TO	fourth
frame of reference	TRY TO CUT	
framework	TRY TO CUT	

function [the verb]	TRY	act, live, work, operate
(is a) function of	CHANGE TO	depends on
fund [the verb]	CHANGE TO	pay for
fundamental	CHANGE TO	basic
funding	TRY	money, paying for
funds	CHANGE TO	money
further [of time or direction]	COMPARE	farther [of distance]

See the comments under *farther*.

furthermore	TRY	and

The introductory *furthermore* should be near the end of the queue of conjunctions that link sentences: after *and*, *in addition*, and *moreover*.

(will in the) future	CHANGE TO	will

G	G	G
give an indication of	CHANGE TO	indicate
give treatment	CHANGE TO	treat
Given . . .	TRY	In, Under, Because of
(the figures) given in the table	CHANGE TO	the figures in the table
(a) given piece of	CHANGE TO	a piece of

H	H	H
(a) half an hour	CHANGE TO	half an hour, a half hour
half of all the ~	CHANGE TO	half the ~
(On the other) hand, . . .	TRY	But . . .
have an effect on	CHANGE TO	affect
have an impact on	CHANGE TO	affect
have got to	CHANGE TO	must
(houses) having	TRY	houses that have
he himself	CHANGE TO	he
(people) having	TRY	people who have
healthful [of food or climate]	COMPARE	healthy [of person or animal]

healthy [of person or animal]	COMPARE	healthful [of food or climate]
help make evident	CHANGE TO	make evident
(be) helpful	CHANGE TO	help
hence	TRY	so, thus, therefore
henceforth	CHANGE TO	from now
her	COMPARE	their

To avoid possible sexist references, the easy solution is to
change the pronoun from singular *(her)* to plural *(their)*,
making sure that the antecedent and the verb number are
changed, too.

her [of a country]	CHANGE TO	its
her(s) and	CHANGE TO	her, and hers

The problem is with a compound possessive.
Hers and Dr. Boynton's gorilla photographs is wrong.
Her and Dr. Boynton's gorilla photographs
is correct but inelegant.
Her gorilla photographs and Dr. Boynton's and *Dr. Boynton's
gorilla photographs and hers* are the solutions.

hereby	CUT OR CHANGE TO	now
herein	CUT OR CHANGE TO	here, in this
hereinafter	CHANGE TO	after this
hereof	CUT	
hereto	CUT	
heretofore	CHANGE TO	until now
herewith	CUT OR CHANGE TO	with this
(by) herself	CHANGE TO	alone
(she) herself	CHANGE TO	she
highly unlikely	CHANGE TO	unlikely
(by) himself	CHANGE TO	alone
(he) himself	CHANGE TO	he
his	COMPARE	their

To avoid possible sexist references, the easy solution is to
change the pronoun from singular *(his)* to plural *(their)*,
making sure that the antecedent and the verb number are
changed, too.

his and	CHANGE TO	his, and his

The problem is with a compound possessive. *His and Dr. Boynton's gorilla photographs* is correct but inelegant. *His gorilla photographs and Dr. Boynton's* and *Dr. Boynton's gorilla photographs and his* are the solutions.

historic [memorable]	COMPARE	historical [of history]
(an) historic	CHANGE TO	a historic

Before *h*, the preference is to use *a* if the *h* is voiced, as in *a hotel*, and *an* if it is not, as in *an hour*.

hitherto	CHANGE TO	until now, until then
hopefully	CUT	
(But +) however	CHANGE TO	But, however
However, it is going to	CHANGE TO	But it is going to; It is, however, going to
humans	CHANGE TO	human beings, people

I	I	I
I	COMPARE	we

Do not write *we* if you mean *I*. *In this book we will show* should be *In this book I will show* if there is one author.

i.e. [that is]	COMPARE	e.g. [for example]
i.e. [*id est* = that is]	CHANGE TO	that is
ideally	TRY TO CUT OR TRY	preferably
identical to	CHANGE TO	identical with, the same as
idiosyncrasies	CHANGE TO	idiosyncrasy, peculiarities
if	COMPARE	though

Some writers put an *if* where a *though* is conventional (and preferred): *a cogent statement, if distorted; a cogent statement, though distorted.*
Such use of *if* should be avoided because it can change the meaning or give two meanings.

If should be reserved for introducing a subordinate clause in a conditional sentence: *If writers followed this principle, there would be less confusion.*

if	COMPARE	whether

If should be reserved for introducing a subordinate clause in a conditional sentence: *If writers followed this principle, there would be less confusion.*
Do not use *if* for *whether: Tell me if you will be going* should be *Tell me whether you will be going.*

If . . . , then . . .	CHANGE TO	If . . . , . . .
if and when	CHANGE TO	if [possibility], when [temporality]
illusion [visual deception or false perception]	COMPARE	allusion [indirect reference], delusion [deception of belief]
immerse with	CHANGE TO	immerse in
immigrate from	CHANGE TO	immigrate to
impact [the noun]	CHANGE TO	effect

The word *impact* should be reserved for its literal meaning: *the impact of the stone on the ground.* If the meaning is figurative—as in *the impact of the program on the population—effect* is preferred. The figurative use of impact is acceptable when writing about the effect of effects, writing that usually deserves rewriting.

impact [the verb]	CHANGE TO	have an effect

Impact is not a verb.

(have an) impact on	CHANGE TO	affect
impede	TRY	stop, hamper, hinder, slow down
(it is) imperative that you	CHANGE TO	you must
implant with	CHANGE TO	implant into
implement	TRY	fulfill, carry out, put into effect
imply [suggest]	COMPARE	infer [conclude]
(is of) importance	CHANGE TO	is important

(More) importantly . . .	CHANGE TO	More important . . .
impracticable [of partic- ular acts or things]	COMPARE	impractical or unpracti- cal [of general actions or things]
impractical [of general actions or things]	COMPARE	impracticable [of partic- ular acts or things]
impressed with	COMPARE	impressed by

A thing is *impressed with* something else; a person is
impressed by someone or something, unless physically
impressed with something.

(located) in	CHANGE TO	in
in ~ terms	CHANGE TO	~ly
in accordance with	CHANGE TO	by, under, in accord with
in addition	TRY	and, also
in addition to	CHANGE TO	besides
in an effort to	CHANGE TO	to
in cases in which	CHANGE TO	if, when
in comparison to	CHANGE TO	in comparison with
in connection with	CHANGE TO	on, for, about
in contrast with	CHANGE TO	in contrast to
in depth	TRY TO CUT OR TRY	~ deep
in excess of	CHANGE TO	more than
in instances in which	CHANGE TO	if, when
(~) in length	CHANGE TO	~ long
in light of	CHANGE TO	in the light of
in order to ~	CHANGE TO	to ~

The exception is in a sentence that has many *to*'s, giving
rise to the need to distinguish the lead infinitive from other
infinitives and from prepositions.
For example: *She had to go to town (in order) to go to the bank*
to get some money.
But even in this sentence, *in order* can be taken out.
If it cannot be taken from a sentence, the sentence should
probably be rewritten.

in order that X might	TRY	for X to
in particular	CUT	
(the ~) in question	CHANGE TO	the ~, this ~, that ~

in regard to	CHANGE TO	on, about
in relation to	TRY	on, about
in respect to	CHANGE TO	on, about
in spite of	CHANGE TO	despite
in spite of the fact that	CHANGE TO	though, although
in support of	CHANGE TO	to, for
in terms of	TRY	as, at, by, in, of, for, with, under, through

The phrase creeps into too many sentences. It should be
replaced by one of the words on the right-hand side.
If that does not work, try rewriting the sentence.

in that	TRY	because
in that case	TRY	then
in the case of	TRY	by, of, in, for
in the event that	CHANGE TO	if
in the field of	CHANGE TO	in
in the final (last) analy- sis	CUT	
(was) in the form of ~	CHANGE TO	was ~
(will) in the future	CHANGE TO	will
in the near future	CHANGE TO	soon
in the neighborhood of	TRY	about
in the past was	CHANGE TO	was
in the region of	CHANGE TO	near, about, close to
in the vicinity of	CHANGE TO	near, about, close to
in the way of	TRY	in
in this connection	CHANGE TO	about
in toto	CHANGE TO	totally, completely, en- tirely
in view of	TRY	because
in view of the fact that	CHANGE TO	because
(~) in width	CHANGE TO	~ wide
in~	COMPARE	un~, non~, not

Tacking *non* on the front of a word is the easiest and sloppi-
est way to make an antonym.
First, try a true antonym: *obscure* to *clear.*
Second, try an antonym created by the prefixes *in* and *un:*
unclear to *clear; insubstantial* to *substantial.*
Third, try *not: not clear* to *clear; not accompanied*
to *accompanied.*

Fourth, having exhausted these possibilities, use *non*.
If the prefix *non* must stand, there should be no hyphen:
non-essential should be *nonessential*. The exception is when
non precedes a capitalized word or a hyphenated construction: *non-English-speaking people*.

inasmuch as	CHANGE TO	because
include [some parts]	COMPARE	comprise [all parts]
included in	CHANGE TO	in
increase [the noun or intransitive verb]	TRY	rise
incredible [hard to believe]	COMPARE	incredulous [skeptical]

Things, events, and actions can be *incredible* to people; only
people can be *incredulous* about something.

incredulous [skeptical]	COMPARE	incredible [hard to be- lieve]

See the comments under *incredible*.

inculcate with	CHANGE TO	inculcate in or into
indebtedness	CHANGE TO	debt
indeed	TRY TO CUT	
independent from	CHANGE TO	independent of
independently	CHANGE TO	on its own, on their own
independently of	CHANGE TO	independent of
indicate	TRY	say, show, suggest
indication	TRY	sign
(is) indicative of	TRY	indicates
indicia	CHANGE TO	signs
individual	TRY	person
individual projects	CHANGE TO	projects
inevitably	CUT	
infer [conclude]	COMPARE	imply [suggest]
infinitely more	CHANGE TO	much more
inflict with	CHANGE TO	inflict on
inform	CHANGE TO	tell, write
infringe on (upon)	CHANGE TO	infringe [violate]
ingenious [clever]	COMPARE	ingenuous [naive, natu- ral]
ingenuous [naive, natu- ral]	COMPARE	ingenious [clever]

inherent in	CHANGE TO	in
initial	TRY	first
initially	TRY	at first
initiate	CHANGE TO	start or begin
inject with	CHANGE TO	inject into
inquire	CHANGE TO	ask
inside of [the preposition]	CHANGE TO	inside
insight into	TRY	idea about
insofar as [= because]	TRY	because
insofar as [= to the extent that]	TRY	so far as
Insofar as ~ is concerned,	CHANGE TO	In, Of, On, For, or About ~,
insoluble [of substances or problems]	COMPARE	unsolvable [of problems]
(for) instance	COMPARE	for example

See the comments under *example*.

(in) instances in which	CHANGE TO	if, when
(in most) instances ~	TRY	most ~s
instead of ~	CHANGE TO	rather than ~
instill with	CHANGE TO	instill into
institute [the verb]	CHANGE TO	start or set up
(was) instrumental in ~ing	CHANGE TO	helped ~
(will be) instrumental in ~ing	CHANGE TO	will help ~
insufficient	TRY	not enough
insure [something]	COMPARE	assure [someone that], ensure [that]
integral part	TRY	part
integrate	TRY	mix, join, combine, amalgamate
integrate into	CHANGE TO	integrate with
intense	COMPARE	intensive

Close in meaning, the two words are often misused as synonyms. The distinction that sometimes helps is to reserve *intense* for passive things, *intensive* for active things: something is *intense*, something applied is *intensive*.
Thus: *War is intense*, but *bombing is intensive*.

The considerable overlap in usage blurs the distinction,
however.

intensive	COMPARE	intense
inter alia [= among others]	CHANGE TO	among others
interface	CHANGE TO	cooperate, work together (unless writing about systems)
into	TRY	in
investigation into	CHANGE TO	investigation of
investments	TRY	investment
involve [a word to avoid]	TRY TO CUT	

The word should seldom replace or be combined with a
preposition. *The government agencies involved in carrying out*
should usually be *this kind of problem* or *these kinds of prob-
involving several departments* should be *The policies of several
departments.* If a verb or participle must stand, try to find a
more precise word, such as *mean, affect,* or *include.*

(the costs) involved in ~	TRY	the cost of ~
irregardless	CHANGE TO	regardless
is	COMPARE	are

See the comments under *are.*

is because	CHANGE TO	is that, is caused by
(in) isolation	CUT OR CHANGE TO	alone
it	TRY TO CUT	

The presence of *it* in a sentence is a signal to look for problems: having two *it*'s referring to more than one antecedent;
having no obvious antecedent; having a wordy construction
that serves little purpose, such as those that follow.

It appears that . . .	CUT
It can be stated with certainty that . . .	CUT
It goes without saying that . . .	CUT

It is apparent that . . .	CUT	
It is important to note that . . .	CUT	
It is to be hoped that . . .	CHANGE TO	I hope . . .
It is ~ that is . . .	CHANGE TO	~ is . . .
It is ~ which is . . .	CHANGE TO	~ is . . .
It should be noted that . . .	CUT	
It should be pointed out that . . .	CUT	
It will be noted that . . .	CUT	
It would appear that . . .	CUT	
its	COMPARE	it's

People still confuse the contraction *it's* (it is) and the possessive *its* (*its'* is not a word).

(by) itself	CHANGE TO	alone
(the ~) itself	CHANGE TO	the ~
-ize [avoid, as in prioritize]	TRY TO CUT	

J   J   J

join together	CHANGE TO	join
judicial [of courts]	COMPARE	judicious [of wisdom]
judicious [of wisdom]	COMPARE	judicial [of courts]
(at this or that) juncture	CHANGE TO	now, then

K   K   K

key [the adjective, a word to avoid]	TRY TO CUT OR TRY	main, important

The word *key* is defensible if it is for opening a real or metaphorical lock.

(is the) key	TRY	is important
(these or those) kinds of ~s	CHANGE TO	this kind of ~, these kinds of ~, that kind of ~, those kinds of ~

The plural is often unnecessary: *these kinds of problems* should usually be *this kind of problems* or *these kinds of problem; those kinds of problems* should usually be *that kind of problem* or *those kinds of problem*.

Some editors prefer to rescue the noun from the prepositional phrase by writing *problems of this (or that) kind*.

L	**L**	**L**
(a) large part of	CHANGE TO	many
(a) large percentage of	CHANGE TO	many
(a) large proportion of	CHANGE TO	many
large-sized ~	TRY	large ~
later on	TRY	later
latter [the adjective as noun]	TRY	last, second

See the comments under *former*.

latter half	TRY	second half
latter part	TRY	later part
laudable [worthy of praise]	COMPARE	laudatory [expressing praise]
laudatory [expressing praise]	COMPARE	laudable [worthy of praise]
lay [put to rest]	COMPARE	lie [be at or come to rest]

Problems arise with the past tense and past participle.
For *lay*, the past tense and participle is *laid*.
Thus: *I think I laid the flowers on the table yesterday, but I could have laid them there the day before.*
For *lie*, the past tense is *lay*, the past participle *lain*.
Thus: *The flowers lay on the table until I picked them up; they could have lain there forever.*

lay out [the verb]	TRY	lay
led to increased competition	CHANGE TO	increased the competition
(~ in) length	CHANGE TO	~ long
lengthy	CHANGE TO	long
less (than) [= a smaller amount of]	COMPARE	fewer (than) [= a smaller number of]

See the comments under *fewer*.

| (the) level of ~ | CHANGE TO | the ~ |

Unless writing about a liquid or hierarchy, try to cut *level:*
the spending is better than *the level of spending; the local peo-*
ple is better than *the people at the local level.*

liable	TRY	likely
licence	CHANGE TO	license
lie [be at or come to rest]	COMPARE	lay [put to rest]

See the comments under *lay.*

| (in) lieu of | CHANGE TO | rather than |
| like | COMPARE | as, as if, such as |

See the comments under *as.*

likely	TRY	probable (probably)
likewise	CHANGE TO	so, also
limitation	TRY	limit
limited	TRY	few, small, meager
linkage	CHANGE TO	link
literal [exact]	COMPARE	figurative [metaphorical]
literally	TRY TO CUT	
loan [the verb]	CHANGE TO	lend
locality (location)	TRY	place
locate	TRY	find
located at (or in)	CHANGE TO	at, in
lose out on	CHANGE TO	lose
(a) lot of	TRY	much, many
loth	CHANGE TO	loath
lots of	TRY	much, many
luxuriant [abundant]	COMPARE	luxurious [of luxury]
luxurious [of luxury]	COMPARE	luxuriant [abundant]

M	**M**	**M**
(decisions) made by	CHANGE TO	decisions by
made up out of	CHANGE TO	made of
magnitude	TRY	size
(the) magnitude of ~	CHANGE TO	the ~

major [= great, greater]	TRY	big, main, chief, great, important, principal
(the) majority of	CHANGE TO	many, most, most of
make a decision about	CHANGE TO	decide about
make changes	CHANGE TO	change
male [the noun]	TRY	man
many of the ~	TRY	many ~
marginal	COMPARE	small

Do not use *marginal* if you mean *small*. *Marginal* refers to increments at the margin or to something at a dividing line.

marginally	CHANGE TO	slightly
masterful [strong-willed]	COMPARE	masterly [skillful]
masterly [skillful]	COMPARE	masterful [strong-willed]
match up	CHANGE TO	match
maximal	TRY	big, high, large, most
maximize [= make most]	TRY	raise, increase
(is) maximized	CHANGE TO	is most, is greatest
maximum [= the most]	TRY	much, most, greatest
may [permission]	COMPARE	can [ability], might [possibility]
may possibly	CHANGE TO	may, might, could
meaningful	CUT	
means	TRY	way
(by) means of	TRY	by
means to produce	CHANGE TO	means of producing, way to produce
media is	CHANGE TO	media are
medium [the adjective]	COMPARE	medium-size

One tendency is to equate *medium* with *small* and *large*; *small and medium firms* should be *small and medium-size firms*; *medium-size and large-size firms* should be *large and medium-size firms*.

methodology [study of method]	COMPARE	method [way to do something]
might [possibility]	COMPARE	can [ability], may [permission]
might possibly	CHANGE TO	might, could
minimal [= the least possible]	TRY	low, small, little, least

minimize [= make least]	TRY	lower, reduce, decrease
(is) minimized	CHANGE TO	is least, lowest, smallest
minimum [= least]	TRY	least, little, lowest, smallest
minor [= small]	TRY	small, unimportant
(the) minority of	TRY	few, some
miss out on	CHANGE TO	miss
mitigate against	CHANGE TO	militate against [make unlikely] or mitigate [reduce]
mode	CHANGE TO	way, method
modicum	CHANGE TO	some
modus	CHANGE TO	way of
moneys	CHANGE TO	money
more substantial	CHANGE TO	greater
more than [for an amount]	COMPARE	over [for a position]

Write *over the table* or *over the moon,* but *more than a dollar, more than 20 percent,* and *more than five hundred years.*

motivate	TRY	make, cause
motivation	TRY	reason
multitude of ~s	TRY	many (or several) ~s
must inevitably	CHANGE TO	must
must necessarily	CHANGE TO	must
mutual [reciprocated]	COMPARE	common [of many]
my (mine) and	CHANGE TO	my, and mine

The problem is with a compound possessive.
Mine and Dr. Boynton's gorilla photographs is wrong.
My and Dr. Boynton's gorilla photographs is correct but inelegant.
My gorilla photographs and Dr. Boynton's
and
Dr. Boynton's gorilla photographs and mine are the solutions.

N   N   N

namely	CUT	
nature [a word to avoid]	TRY TO CUT	

As with *case* and *character*, the word is best avoided. Here
are the most common abuses and the ways around them:
the secret nature of should be *the secrecy of;*
the nature of the work is secret and *the work is of a secret
nature* should be *the work is secret* or *the secrecy of the work.*

(is of a ~) nature	CHANGE TO	is ~
(in the) near future	TRY	soon
necessarily	TRY TO CUT	
necessary	TRY	needed
necessitate	TRY	need, require
necessity	TRY	need, requirement
needless to say	CUT	
(in the) negative	CHANGE TO	no
(in the) neighborhood of [= about]	CHANGE TO	about
neither a, b, nor c	CHANGE TO	Of a, b, and c, none . . .

Many editors dislike the use of *neither-nor* with more than
two elements. There naturally are some outstanding exceptions: *Neither rain, sleet, snow, and so on.*

neither of them are	CHANGE TO	neither of them is
never the less	CHANGE TO	nevertheless
nevertheless	COMPARE	nonetheless

Take your pick and stick to it.

no doubt	TRY TO CUT	
non~	TRY	in~, un~, not

See the comments under *in~*.

none	COMPARE	not one

The decision to use one or the other turns on whether
emphasis is wanted: *not one* is more emphatic than *none*.

none of them are	CHANGE TO	none of them is
none the less	CHANGE TO	nonetheless
nor	COMPARE	or

Nor is acceptable as the correlative conjunction with *neither*
or at the beginning of a negative sentence that follows a
negative sentence: *They did not go to the beach. Nor did they
go to the mountains.*
Many people incorrectly use *nor* as a conjunction after a
negative verb: *They did not go to the beach nor the mountains.*
Or should replace *nor* in the example.

not a	TRY	no
not . . . nor	CHANGE TO	not . . . or
not only . . . , but also	TRY TO CUT OR TRY	not only . . . , but . . .

Much overused as correlative conjunctions, *not only* and *but
also* should be used sparingly and only with compound
sentences. *The concert was not only long, but also boring*
should be either *The concert was long and boring* or *Not only
was the concert long; it was boring.* These correlatives are also
a favorite in sentences that begin with *It: It is not only
unsurprising, but also expected, that* could just as easily
be *It is unsurprising, even expected, that* which could
even be *It is expected that.*

not the same	CHANGE TO	different
not un~	CHANGE TO	~

Recall Orwell's complaint:
*A not unblack dog was chasing a not unsmall rabbit across a not
ungreen field.*

notwithstanding	TRY	despite
number [a word to avoid]	TRY TO CUT	
(a) number of	CUT OR CHANGE TO	some, many, several, forty-three

Improve such constructions as *a number of firms* by writing
some firms, many firms, several firms, or *forty-three* firms. If it
is not possible to be more precise, simply write *firms.*
Change such constructions as *ten times the number of jobs* to
ten times the jobs.

Overall,	TRY TO CUT	
overall	COMPARE	whole, total, entire, average, aggregate
(the) overall ~	TRY	the ~
overly	CHANGE TO	too, too much
owing to	TRY	caused by, because of
owing to the fact that	CHANGE TO	because
own [the adjective]	TRY TO CUT	

His own car should be *his car*.

P	**P**	**P**
parameter	TRY	limit, boundary, condition
(a large) part of	CHANGE TO	much, many
(a small) part of	CHANGE TO	some
(on the) part of	TRY	by, of, from
partake in	CHANGE TO	partake of
partially	TRY	partly
(this or that) particular ~	CHANGE TO	this (or that) ~
party	TRY	person
(in the) past was	TRY	was
(to) pay off	CHANGE TO	to pay, to repay
pending	TRY	until
people [in general]	COMPARE	persons [in particular]
per	TRY	a

Barrels per day or *barrels a day; dollars per year* or *dollars a year; GNP per person* or *GNP a person; rate per hour* or *rate an hour.*
Many writers use *per* all the time; some editors push for using *a* (*an*) all the time. The best practice probably is to use *a much of the time* and to resort to *per* if *a* sounds unnatural.

(as) per	CHANGE TO	on, for, about, further to, in accord with
per se	CUT	
percent of ~	CHANGE TO	percentage of ~, proportion of ~
(a) percentage of	CHANGE TO	part of

(a large) percentage of	CHANGE TO	much, many
(a small) percentage of	CHANGE TO	some
period of time	CHANGE TO	time, period
(over a) period of three years	CHANGE TO	over three years
persons [in particular]	COMPARE	people [in general]
persuade [someone of, to, or that]	COMPARE	convince [someone to or that]

There is much overlap except before *to,* where only *persuade* will do. See the comments under *convince.*

pertaining to	CHANGE TO	about
pertains to	CHANGE TO	is about
peruse	CHANGE TO	read
(this) phenomena	CHANGE TO	this phenomenon
(at this) point in time	CHANGE TO	now, at this point, at this time
(from the) point of view of ~	CHANGE TO	for ~
portion	CHANGE TO	part
posterior to	CHANGE TO	after
potential [the noun]	TRY TO CUT	
potential gains	TRY	possible gains
practicable [of particular acts or things]	COMPARE	practical [of general actions or things]
practical [of general actions or things]	COMPARE	practicable [of particular acts or things]
practically	CHANGE TO	almost, nearly
pre- [as in preprocessing]	CHANGE TO	before processing
preceding [the one just passed]	COMPARE	previous [past]
precipitate [rash, abrupt]	COMPARE	precipitous [steep]
precipitous [steep]	COMPARE	precipitate [rash, abrupt]
predicated on	CHANGE TO	based on
predominant(ly)	TRY	main(ly) or chief(ly)
prefer ~ over	CHANGE TO	prefer ~ to
preferable	CHANGE TO	best, better, preferred
preliminary to	CHANGE TO	before
preparatory to	CHANGE TO	before
(is) prepared to	CHANGE TO	is ready (or willing) to

prescribe [dictate or ordain]	COMPARE	proscribe [outlaw or prohibit]
(at) present	CHANGE TO	now
(the) present ~	CHANGE TO	this ~

The seeming need for *present* comes from the requirement to distinguish, say, two other books from this one, unnecessarily called *the present book*.

(the) present writer	CHANGE TO	I
presented in this ~	CHANGE TO	in this ~
presently	CHANGE TO	now, soon
pressures	TRY	pressure
pretty [the weak intensifier]	CUT	
preventative	CHANGE TO	preventive
previous [past]	COMPARE	preceding [the one just passed]
previous to	CHANGE TO	before
previously	CHANGE TO	before, earlier
(have) previously received	CHANGE TO	have received
principal(ly)	TRY	main(ly) or chief(ly)
prior [the adjective]	TRY	earlier
prior experience	CHANGE TO	experience
prior to	CHANGE TO	before
prioritize [and similar obscenities]	CHANGE TO	set priorities for
priority [a word to avoid]	TRY TO CUT	
proceed	CHANGE TO	go, go ahead
process [a word to avoid]	TRY TO CUT	
(the) process of, say, modernization	CHANGE TO	modernization
(the decision-making) process	CHANGE TO	decision-making
procure	CHANGE TO	get
pronounced [the adjective]	CHANGE TO	great
proper	TRY TO CUT	
prophecy [the noun]	COMPARE	prophesy [the verb]
prophesy [the verb]	COMPARE	prophecy [the noun]
proportion	CHANGE TO	part

(a large) proportion of	CHANGE TO	much, many
(a small) proportion of	CHANGE TO	some
(the greater) proportion of	CHANGE TO	most
proscribe [outlaw or prohibit]	COMPARE	prescribe [dictate or ordain]
proven	TRY	proved

The past tense and past participle of *prove* is *proved* not
proven, but *proven* has invaded the place of *proved* in
speech, and thus in much writing: *until proven guilty;
proven oil reserves.*
Proved is the correct word in both examples.

provide	TRY	give, have, offer
provide a summary	COMPARE	summarize

A person *provides a summary* by handing or sending one to
another person. A person (or introduction or conclusion)
summarizes by drawing the main points together for an
audience or reader.

provided (providing) that	TRY	if

The change should always be made in introductory clauses
of stipulation: *Provided (that) she goes* should be *If she goes.*

(in close) proximity to	CHANGE TO	near, close to
purchase [the verb]	CHANGE TO	buy
(for the) purpose of	CHANGE TO	for
(for the) purpose of ~ing	CHANGE TO	to ~

For the purpose of getting to work on time should be *To get to
work on time.*

(with the) purpose of ~ing	CHANGE TO	to ~
pursue	TRY	follow

Q	Q	Q
qua	CHANGE TO	as
quasi-money	CHANGE TO	quasi money
quasi public body	CHANGE TO	quasi-public body
(the ~ in) question	CHANGE TO	the ~, this ~, that ~,
(the) question of whether	CHANGE TO	whether, the question whether
quite	CUT	
quote [as a noun]	CHANGE TO	quotation

Quote is a verb, not a noun: *The quote is from a column by William Raspberry* should be *The quotation is from a column by William Raspberry.*

R	R	R
rapidity	CHANGE TO	speed
(but) rather	CHANGE TO	but
Rather, . . .	CHANGE TO	Instead, . . .
rather [the modifier]	CUT	
rationale	TRY	plan, reason, thinking
re	CUT OR CHANGE TO	about
reach a conclusion	CHANGE TO	conclude
(the conclusion) reached	CHANGE TO	the conclusion
reaction	TRY	response, impression
real	TRY TO CUT	
(the) reason is because	CHANGE TO	the reason is that
(by) reason of	CHANGE TO	because of
(for the) reason that	CHANGE TO	because, since
(the) reason why	TRY	the reason, the reason that, the reason for ~ to be
receive	TRY	get, have
(is the) recipient of	CHANGE TO	got
redolent with	CHANGE TO	redolent of
reduce (reduction)	TRY	try
refer [directly]	COMPARE	allude [refer indirectly]

refer back	CHANGE TO	refer
(with) reference to	CHANGE TO	of, on, for, about
reflect	TRY	show
(in) regard to	CHANGE TO	on, about
(with) regard to	CHANGE TO	of, on, for, about
regarding	TRY	on, for, about
(as) regards	CHANGE TO	on, for, about
(in the) region of	CHANGE TO	near, about, close to
relate	TRY	say, tell
relates to	TRY	of, on, about
related to	TRY	has to do with
relating to	TRY	on, for, about
relation	COMPARE	relationship

Some people use these words as synonyms.
One way to differentiate them is to use them thus: The *relationship* between the United States and Western Europe; East-West *relations;* the *relationship* between two people; a person's *relatives,* not *relations;* the *relation* between exports and gross national product; and so on. There is nothing hard and fast to disentangle usage, except to prefer the shorter word.

(in) relation to	TRY	on, about
relationship	COMPARE	relation

See the comments under *relation*.

relative(ly)	TRY TO CUT	
rely upon	CHANGE TO	rely on
remunerate (remuneration)	CHANGE TO	pay
render	CHANGE TO	give, make
replace	COMPARE	substitute

The prepositions determine the use of these seeming synonyms: *replace X by Y,* not *replace X for Y; substitute X for Y,* not *substitute X by Y.*

replicate	TRY	copy, reproduce
reportedly	CUT	

represents	TRY	is, makes up
require	TRY	need, want, call for
requirement	TRY	need
requisite [the adjective]	CHANGE TO	needed
requisite [the noun]	CHANGE TO	needed thing
reside	TRY	live
(in or with) respect to	CHANGE TO	on, for, about
respective(ly)	TRY TO CUT	

If the links between the elements of a sentence are ambiguous, rewrite it. The most common rewrite is from: *Bob turned fifty and Alice turned forty in 1975 and in 1976, respectively* to *Bob turned fifty in 1975, and Alice turned forty in 1976.*

result in [the verb]	CHANGE TO	lead to

The reasons are that *lead to* saves a syllable and avoids possible confusion with the noun *result*.

(as a) result of	CHANGE TO	from, because of
reveal	TRY	show
revenues	CHANGE TO	revenue
reverse	COMPARE	converse, obverse

See the comments under *converse*.

reverse [back of coin]	COMPARE	obverse [front of coin]
role	TRY TO CUT OR TRY	importance

Many editors feel that *roles* should be reserved for the stage. The standard change is from *The role of the vaccine in eradicating polio* to *The importance of the vaccine in eradicating polio.*
But it is not always that easy.

rose by 2 percent	CHANGE TO	rose 2 percent

This change does not work for fractions.
In *rose by half* the *by* must stand.

S	S	S
~s'	CHANGE TO	~s's
~'s	COMPARE	of ~

The possessive form is fine for people, but if extended, say, to countries, it introduces what Follett calls the false possessive.
Brazil's GNP is an illogical construction because Brazil is incapable of possessing a GNP. The phrase should be rewritten as *the GNP of Brazil*.
Or so the logic goes. The logic nevertheless breaks down with *its*, which is fine as an inanimate possessive: *its population*. The best practice is to avoid false possessives in scholarly writing and to avoid excessive use of false possessives in other writing.

said	COMPARE	wrote, written
(not the) same	CHANGE TO	different
savings	COMPARE	saving

The general preference is to use *savings* as an adjective, *saving* as a noun: *savings accounts* and *savings rates,* but *national saving* and *the rate of saving*. There naturally is a middle ground of confusion, such as with a *family's savings* and *a saving grace*.
But the general preference is worth keeping in mind. So is the idea of trying to make plural nouns singular.

. . . , say, of five years	CHANGE TO	. . . of, say, five years
secondly	CHANGE TO	second
secure [the verb]	CHANGE TO	get
seek	CHANGE TO	try, look for
seem(s)	COMPARE	is, are
semi-detached	CHANGE TO	semidetached

The general preference is to run the prefix *semi* solid. Some editors run it solid only before consonants, hyphenating it before a vowel, as in *semi-industrial*.

semiannually	TRY	twice a year
semimonthly	TRY	twice a month
semiweekly	TRY	twice a week

(will) serve to ~	CHANGE TO	~s
serves to ~	CHANGE TO	~s
set forth	CHANGE TO	give
shall	CHANGE TO	will

Shall can be forgotten in today's writing. But if you want to preserve the distinctions between *shall* and *will*, see Strunk and White.

she [of country]	CHANGE TO	it
she herself	CHANGE TO	she
should	TRY	would
significant [of statistical relations and things signified]	COMPARE	big, large, important
since	COMPARE	because

Some editors, in the interest of not putting readers on the wrong scent, reserve *because* for cause and *since* for time: *Because I am going,* but *Since 1941.* The wrong scent is evident in such a construction as *Since I have been going,* which could relate to cause or to time.

(a) single ~	TRY	one ~
situated in	CHANGE TO	in
skills	TRY	skill
(a) small part of	CHANGE TO	some
(a) small percentage of	CHANGE TO	some
(a) small proportion of	CHANGE TO	some
small-sized	CHANGE TO	small
So	TRY TO CUT	

Useful but often overused as a conjunction.

so as not to ~	CHANGE TO	to ~

The words that fill in the blanks must be opposites, which an example can make clear: *so as not to obscure* is longer than but equal to *to clarify.*

so as to	CHANGE TO	to
so long as	COMPARE	as long as

Purists reserve so long as for negative constructions, as long as for positive: So long as you do not fail but As long as you succeed.

soluble [of substances or problems]	COMPARE	solvable [of problems]
solvable [of problems]	COMPARE	soluble [of substances or problems]
some of the ~	CHANGE TO	some ~s
somewhat	CUT	
sought	CHANGE TO	tried, looked for
specific	TRY TO CUT	

A specific program is usually the same as a program.

(in) spite of	CHANGE TO	despite
(in) spite of the fact that	CHANGE TO	(al)though
stanch [the verb]	COMPARE	staunch [the adjective]
(from the) standpoint of	CHANGE TO	for
start up	TRY	start
starting out with	CHANGE TO	starting with
state [the verb]	CHANGE TO	say
staunch [the adjective]	COMPARE	stanch [the verb]
(will take) steps to ~	CHANGE TO	will ~
strategy	TRY	plan
(to) subject to tax	CHANGE TO	to tax
(is) subjected to tax	CHANGE TO	is taxed

The formula is to cut subject(ed) to and to change the noun to a verb. It does not always work.

subsequent	CHANGE TO	later
subsequent to	CHANGE TO	after
subsequently	CHANGE TO	later, then
substitute	COMPARE	replace

The prepositions determine the use of these seeming synonyms: replace X by Y, not replace X for Y; substitute X for Y, not substitute X by Y.

such as	COMPARE	like

See the comments under *as*.

(~s,) such as . . .	TRY	such ~s as . . .

This change can do away with two commas and improve cadence, but it cannot always be made.

Leading oil companies, such as Exxon, Mobil, and British Petroleum, are . . . could be written *Such leading oil companies as Exxon, Mobil, and British Petroleum are.* . . .

The change seems to work best if the noun exemplified is general and not specific, worst if the noun is particular, preceded by *the*.

such as X, Y, Z, and so on	CHANGE TO	such as X, Y, and Z
(on) such factors as ~	TRY	on, say, ~
(until) such time as	CHANGE TO	until
sufficient(ly)	TRY	enough
(the) sum of $1 million	CHANGE TO	$1 million
(in) support of	CHANGE TO	to, for
supposing (supposing that)	CHANGE TO	if

T   **T**   **T**

take account of	COMPARE	take into account

Use one or the other.

take action	CHANGE TO	act
take into account	COMPARE	take account of

Use one or the other.

(will) take steps to	CHANGE TO	will
(both facts) taken together	CHANGE TO	both facts
(is) tantamount to	CHANGE TO	means
target [a word to avoid]	TRY	aim, goal, objective
(have a) tendency to	CHANGE TO	tend to
terminate	TRY	end
termination	TRY	ending
(in) ~ terms	TRY	~ly

| (in) terms of | TRY | by, in, of, for, with, under, through, in relation to |

The construction should seldom be permitted to stand.
In terms of value added should be *In value added*.
Explain in terms of should be *Explain by*.
Another way around *in terms of* is rewriting.

| thankfully | CUT | |
| that | COMPARE | which |

The important things are knowing why you use one or
the other and punctuating *which* clauses correctly.
See chapter 7.

| that is (are) | TRY TO CUT |

Try to delete *that is (are)* in a restrictive clause: *An item that is
exported* is the same as but longer than *An item exported*.
The same goes for *Factors that are deleterious to*, which can
be cut to *Factors deleterious to*.

| the [particular] | COMPARE | a, an [general] |

See the comments under *a, an*.

| the ~ of | TRY | ~ing |

The phrase *the manufacture of* can almost always be changed
to *manufacturing, the production of* to *producing*. The same
goes in spades for *the manufacturing of* and *the producing of*.

| the fact that | TRY | that |
| their(s) and | CHANGE TO | their, and theirs |

The problem is with a compound possessive.
Theirs and Dr. Boynton's gorilla photographs is wrong.
Their and Dr. Boynton's gorilla photographs is correct but
inelegant.
Their gorilla photographs and Dr. Boynton's
and
Dr. Boynton's gorilla photographs and theirs are the solutions.

(by) themselves	TRY	alone
(the ~s) themselves	CHANGE TO	the ~s
There are big differences	CHANGE TO	Differences are big

This is one of the most common changes by editors. The formula, with a *There are* opening followed by an adjective and noun, is to pull the noun ahead of the verb to replace *There*.

there are now	CHANGE TO	there are

The tense of the verb usually is enough to indicate time and to make the adverb redundant.
The same thing happens with *there were in the past* and *there will be in the future.*
But not with *yesterday, today,* and *tomorrow* if they refer to days.

there exist	CHANGE TO	there are
thereafter	CHANGE TO	then, after that
thereby	CHANGE TO	by it, by that

Better still, change the construction from passive to active through rewriting: from *the changes indicated thereby* to *the changes indicated by it* to *the changes it indicates.*
Two birds, one stone.

therefor	CHANGE TO	for it
therefore	TRY	thus
therefrom	CHANGE TO	from it
therein	CHANGE TO	there, in it
thereof	CHANGE TO	its, of it
thereto	CHANGE TO	to it, about it
thereupon	CHANGE TO	then
therewith	CHANGE TO	with it
these kinds of ~s	CHANGE TO	this kind of ~, these kinds of ~

The plural is often unnecessary: *these kinds of problems* should usually be *this kind of problem* or *these kinds of problem.* Some editors prefer to rescue the noun from the prepositional phrase by writing *problems of this kind.*

think [for speculations]	COMPARE	feel [for emotions], believe [for convictions]
thirdly	CHANGE TO	third
This . . .	COMPARE	The . . .

It often happens in consecutive sentences that the subject of
one is, say, *This distinction* or *That* referring to the distinction. What is to be done if the subject of the next sentence
is the same? *This distinction* would be repetitive, which is
not bad. *That* would be ambiguous, which is bad. Clear and
elegant, however, is *The distinction*, more so than *Such a
distinction*, which is another possibility.

this (that) particular ~	CHANGE TO	this (that) ~
thorough	CUT	
those ~ in which	CHANGE TO	~ which
those ~ that	CHANGE TO	~ that, those that

Those restricts the noun it precedes, just as a *that* clause
restricts the noun it follows. To use both is to be doubly
restrictive, which is not necessary.
The solution is to cut *those* or to cut the noun and have the
adjective as a substantive pronoun:
those bundles of kindling that we sold
should be
(the) bundles of kindling that we sold
or
those that we sold, if the noun is clear.

those kinds of ~s	CHANGE TO	that kind of ~, those kinds of ~

The plural is often unnecessary: *those kinds of problems*
should usually be *that kind of problem* or *those kinds of problem*. Some editors prefer to rescue the noun from a prepositional phrase by writing *problems of that kind*.

those people who	CHANGE TO	those who, people who

As with *those* and *that*, to use both *those* and *who* is to be
doubly restrictive.

The solution is to cut *those* or to cut the noun and have the
adjective as a substantive pronoun:
those people who went should be *(the) people who went* or
those who went, if the noun is clear.

| though | COMPARE | although |
| though | COMPARE | if |

See the comments under *if.*

| thus | COMPARE | therefore |
| thus | TRY | so |

At the beginning of a sentence, *so* is less formal than *thus* or
therefore. Keep in mind, however, that *so* is often overused
as a conjunction.

thusly	CHANGE TO	thus
(at that point in) time	CHANGE TO	then, at that time, at that point
(at this point in) time	CHANGE TO	now, at this time, at this point
(changes over) time	CHANGE TO	changes
time period	CHANGE TO	time, period
(period of) time	CHANGE TO	time, period
(at the) time when	CHANGE TO	when
to + adverb + verb	TRY	to + verb, adverb + to + verb, to + verb + adverb

Seldom split an infinitive: *to needlessly split an infinitive*
should be *to split an infinitive needlessly, needlessly to split an
infinitive,* or simply *to split an infinitive.*
Two uses of the split infinitive are unassailable: if the
adverb is more important than the infinitive, as in *to
blithely go;* if rejoining the infinitive makes a sentence
sound strange.

to try and do	CHANGE TO	to try to do
. . ., to wit:	CHANGE TO	. . . :
together with	CHANGE TO	with
total ~	CHANGE TO	~

toward	COMPARE	to
towards	CHANGE TO	toward

On the western side of the Atlantic, the s has succumbed
to the newspaper editor's pencil.

transmit	TRY	send
transpire [become known]	COMPARE	occur, happen
transportation	CHANGE TO	transport
try out	TRY	try
turbid [muddy]	COMPARE	turgid [swollen]
turgid [swollen]	COMPARE	turbid [muddy]
twice	COMPARE	double

Usage now seems to be to reserve *double* for the verb and
twice for the noun, as in *I'll double what I give you; I'll
give you twice that amount.*

type	TRY	kind
(these or those) types of ~s	CHANGE TO	this type of ~, these types of ~, that type of ~, those types of ~

Note first that *type* should often be *kind.*
Note second that the plural is often unnecessary: *these types
of ships* should usually be *this type of ship* or *these types of
ship.*
Some editors prefer to rescue the noun from the prepositional phrase by writing *ships of this type.*

(oldest ~ of its) type	TRY	oldest ~ of its kind

U	U	U
U.S.	COMPARE	United States

Spell it out, except as an adjective.
U.S. interests but *in the United States.*

ultimate	TRY	last, final
ultimately	TRY	finally, in the end
un~	COMPARE	in~, non~, not

See the comments under *in*~.

| underway | CHANGE TO | under way |

The adjective *underway* is seldom used; the adverb *under way*, as in *construction is under way*, is almost always what is intended by *underway*.

undue (unduly)	CUT	
unpractical [of general actions or things]	COMPARE	impracticable [of particular actions or things]
unfortunately	CUT OR CHANGE TO	but

The word should not be used more than once in a manuscript, if that often, for it adds nothing.

unless and until	CHANGE TO	unless
(highly) unlikely	CHANGE TO	unlikely
unnecessarily	CHANGE TO	needlessly
until such time as	CHANGE TO	until
untimely	CUT	
[rely, depend, or insist] upon	CHANGE TO	rely on, depend on, or insist on
usage	COMPARE	use

Usage refers to a manner of use—rough, for example—or to a habitual practice that creates a standard, as in language. *Use* should be used for all other uses.

| useful | TRY TO CUT | |
| utilize (utilization) | TRY | use |

The scholarly exception is to use *utilize* for use against a standard, as in *capacity utilization*. But *capacity use* conveys just as much.

V	V	V
(a) variety of	CHANGE TO	many several, different
various	TRY TO CUT OR TRY	different
verbal [of words]	COMPARE	oral [of mouth]

versus [= so as to face]	CHANGE TO	against, as against, compared with, in contrast to
very	CUT	
via	CHANGE TO	by, through, by way of
viable [ability to live and grow]	TRY	lasting, practicable, workable
(the) viability of	TRY TO CUT	
(in the) vicinity of	CHANGE TO	near, about, close to
(in) view of	TRY	because
(in) view of the fact that	CHANGE TO	because
(with a) view to ~ing	CHANGE TO	to ~
viewpoint	TRY	view
virtually	CHANGE TO	nearly, almost
virtually all	CHANGE TO	most
(by) virtue of	CHANGE TO	by
vis-à-vis [= face to face with]	TRY	compared with, relative to, in relation to
visualize	TRY	see, think of, imagine
volume [book]	CHANGE TO	book
(the) volume of demand for ~	CHANGE TO	the demand for ~

WXYZ

WXYZ	WXYZ	WXYZ
was	COMPARE	were

See the comments under *are*. For use with the conditional, distinguish past impossibility (if I was) and future possibility (if I were to go).

(in the) way of	TRY	in
(by) way of ~ing	CHANGE TO	to ~
we	COMPARE	I

Do not write *we* if you mean *I*. *In this book we will show*
should be
In this book I will show if there is one author.

(as) well as	TRY	and, also
were	COMPARE	was

See the comments under *are* and *was*.

when	COMPARE	if, in which
when and if	CHANGE TO	if [possibility], when [temporality]
when the ~ was over	CHANGE TO	after the ~
where	COMPARE	if, when, in which
whereas	CHANGE TO	but, though
whereby	CUT OR CHANGE TO	so that
wherein	CHANGE TO	in which
wherewithal	CHANGE TO	means, money
whether	COMPARE	if

See the comments under *if*.

whether or not	CHANGE TO	whether

The *or not* often is not needed:
The managers are trying to decide whether they should adopt the policy (or not). In this and in many other constructions, the *or not* can be dropped.

which	COMPARE	that

The important things are knowing why you use one or the other and punctuating *which* clauses correctly.
See chapter 7.

(of) which	TRY	whose

Whose is a useful word that fills the gap between *who* and *that*, a gap that too often is infelicitously filled by *of which*.

which is (are)	TRY TO CUT	

Try to delete *which is (are)* in a restrictive clause: *An item which is exported* is the same as but longer than *An item exported*. The same goes for *Factors which are deleterious to,* which can be cut to *Factors deleterious to.* Recall that the preference of this book is to reserve *which* for nonrestrictive clauses. Try, too, to delete *which is (are)* in a nonrestrictive clause. Thus: *The plan, which is the first of many, . . .* can be shortened to *The plan, the first of many, . . .*

whichever	TRY TO CUT	
while	TRY	when, although

Some writers follow the practice—and it is a good one—of reserving *while* for clauses describing action at the same time as the principal clause, *although* for clauses describing opposing conditions. If the subordinate clause follows the main clause, *while* is not preceded by a comma.

Thus: *He went to town, while she slept* should be *He went to town while she slept* if the meaning of *while* is *during the time that.* If the meaning is *and,* as in *He went to town, while she slept,* change the comma to a semicolon and cut *while: He went to town; she slept.*

(stay a) while	CHANGE TO	stay awhile

But stay *for a while.*

whilst	CHANGE TO	while
who	COMPARE	whom

It would be nice to settle the confusion in one sentence, but it is not that simple. The basic problem is that the two words are so often confused in speech. The most common errors are using *who* for *whom* at the start of a question, as in *Who did they fire?* and using *whom* for *who* in a nonrestrictive clause, as in *The mayor, whom reporters said would be running for reelection, was silent about his plans. Whom* is correct in the first example, *who* in the second.

who is (are)	TRY TO CUT	

Try to delete *who is (are)* in a restrictive clause: *A person who is going to France* is the same as but longer than *A person going to France.* Try, too, to delete *who is (are)* in a nonrestrictive clause. Thus: *New Yorkers, who are thought by many to be cold, . . .* can be shortened to *New Yorkers, thought by many to be cold, ...*

whole [the adjective]   TRY TO CUT

Many writers unwittingly use *whole* to modify something that is by definition whole: *throughout the whole country* says no more than *throughout the county.*

| whom | COMPARE | who |

See the comments under *who.*

(~ in) width	CHANGE TO	~ wide
will in the future	CHANGE TO	will
will take steps to	CHANGE TO	will
~wise	CHANGE TO	for ~, about ~

Especially in such atrocities as electricitywise.
There are some unexceptionable exceptions:
clockwise, likewise, lengthwise, and
otherwise.

wish	TRY	want
With [in the sense of *Given*]	CHANGE TO	Because of
with a view to ~ing	CHANGE TO	to ~
with reference to	CHANGE TO	of, on, for, about
with regard to	CHANGE TO	of, on, for, about
with respect to	CHANGE TO	on, for, about
with the exception of	CHANGE TO	except
within	TRY	in, between

The change almost always improves a sentence.
Within should be used when the object of the
preposition is an area or space—and as a synonym
for *inside of,* as in limits.

woman [as adjective]	CHANGE TO	female
(in the) year 2000	CHANGE TO	in 2000
you	COMPARE	people

The second person should be used only in giving advice or instructions or in writing a letter or memorandum to someone.

| your(s) and | CHANGE TO | your, and yours |

The problem is with a compound possessive. *Yours and Dr. Boynton's gorilla photographs* is wrong.
Your and Dr. Boynton's gorilla photographs is correct but inelegant. *Your gorilla photographs and Dr. Boynton's* and *Dr. Boynton's gorilla photographs and yours* are the solutions.

Latin Words, Phrases, and Abbreviations

| *a fortiori* [= with even greater force] | CUT OR CHANGE TO | even more, more obviously |
| *a priori* [= from the former] | COMPARE | *prima facie* [= at first view] |

Some confusion arises because of the similarity of some meanings of the two phrases. *A priori* refers to deductive reasoning—from causes or self-evident propositions to effects; in this sense it is the opposite of *a posteriori*. *A priori* also means to be without examination or analysis. In this sense the phrase often is mistakenly used for *prima facie*, which means at first glance. The two phrases can act as adverbs or adjectives.

a priori	TRY	deductive(ly), presumptive(ly)
a posteriori [= from what has been observed]	TRY	inductive(ly)
circa [= around]	CHANGE TO	about, around
ceteris paribus [= other things being equal]	CHANGE TO	other things being equal

cf. [*confer* = com-pare]	CHANGE TO	compare
cum [= with]	CHANGE TO	and, with, com-bined with
e.g. [*exempli gratia* = by way of example]	CHANGE TO	say, for example
e.g. [for example]	COMPARE	i.e. [that is]
et al. [*et alia* = and others]	CHANGE TO	and others
etc. [*et cetera* = and the others]	CHANGE TO	and so on, and so forth
i.e. [*id est* = that is]	CHANGE TO	that is
i.e. [that is]	COMPARE	e.g. [for example]
ibid. [*ibidem* = in the same place]	CHANGE TO	in the same work
inter alia [= among others]	CHANGE TO	among others
ipso facto [= by the fact itself]	CUT OR CHANGE TO	by that fact
mutatis mutandis [= with the changes needed]	CHANGE TO	with the changes needed
n.b. [*nota bene* = note well]	CHANGE TO	note well
non sequitur [= it does not follow]	CHANGE TO	does not follow
op. cit. [*opere citato* = in the work cited]	CHANGE TO	in the work cited
pari passu [= with equal step]	CHANGE TO	at the same time, pace, or rate; hand in hand
passim [= scattered]	CHANGE TO	here and there
prima facie [= at first view]	COMPARE	*a priori* [= from the former]

See the comments under *a priori*.

prima facie [= at first view]	CHANGE TO	at first glance
q.v. [*quod vide* = which see]	CHANGE TO	for which, see . . .
sine qua non [= with-out which not]	CHANGE TO	an essential thing

| v. or vs. [*versus* = against] | CHANGE TO | against, with | compared |
| viz. [*videlicet* = namely] | CUT OR CHANGE TO | | :, that is |

The best solution usually is to replace *viz.*
by a colon.